Helena Smole

Balancing the Beast

A Bright View of Schizoaffective Disorder
—
Bipolar or Manic-Depressive Type

Helena Smole
BALANCING THE BEAST
A Bright View of Schizoaffective Disorder
– Bipolar or Manic-Depressive Type

Illustrations by Leon Zuodar
Cover Design and Typesetting by Miha Bercko
English Language Editing by Dean J. DeVos
Published by:
Bubina Baita, Slovenia, Europe
info@bubinabaita.com

All rights reserved. No part of this book may be reproduced or transmitted in any form or by any means, electronic or mechanical, including photocopying, recording or by any information storage and retrieval system, without written permission from the author, except for the inclusion of brief quotations in a review.

Copyright © 2011 by Helena Smole.

CIP - Kataložni zapis o publikaciji
Narodna in univerzitetna knjižnica, Ljubljana

616.89-008.1

SMOLE, Helena, 1974-
  Balancing the beast : a bright view of schizoaffective
disorder – bipolar or manic-depressive type / Helena Smole ;
[illustrations by Leon Zuodar]. - Ljubljana : Bubina Baita, 2010

ISBN 978-961-92979-0-2

253522432

To you, dear reader.

Blessed are those who can laugh at themselves for they shall never cease to be amused.

(Anonymous)

Why bother?

At first I thought it would be best not to share my thoughts on Helena's experiences with mental illness in her book because I may be too subjective. After all, she has been my spouse for some time now. But then again, who else should answer this "intimate" question: Why bother?

From what I hear now, some people I believed I knew quite well and some people I barely knew, wanted to ask me that question years ago. Why bother? They probably meant why stick with Helena when it was obvious she had serious mental health issues. This was when her third manic-depressive episode occurred and the ordeals reached a peak, at least as far as I was concerned. At those times when we slept at most a few hours a day, while the manic episode was rampant, or when watching her lie in bed all month long probably thinking of committing suicide (although at that time I did not know that she had such thoughts), I could have, at least theoretically, left her just by herself. After all, why bother?

Well, leaving her and thus supposedly making my life easier was not an option. Why not? We had met each other while running a half-marathon. Those who have tried it might agree that running a half-marathon is more than a walk in the park. While running the final miles of the race it was obvious to me that she was having problems. But she persisted. At that moment I realized that she was a fighter, even though I had known her for less than an hour. And, later on, when it became obvious she had mental health issues, it was immensely easier for me to stick with her. Why? She was a fighter in those situations, too.

Besides being prepared to work hard, I think it takes something else to cope well with this kind of mental illness. To us, upon realizing that we would have to live with the obvious negative consequences of this mental illness for the rest of our lives despite Helena taking her prescribed antipsychotic drugs, it looked like a pretty bleak future indeed. Anyway, there was a strong feeling that we would have to change something. Most probably ourselves. And if there was one thing I knew, it is that you cannot change a person if the person is reluctant to change. Helena was prepared to start changing her thinking patterns even though there was no guarantee of a positive outcome at all. This was another reason to stand by her.

Today it seems, at least according to the feedback Helena has received from psychiatrists (see the testimonials, for examples), that the path she chose, in addition to taking pills, was good. However, when reading this book you might be misled into giving me too much credit for Helena's achievements. I sincerely ask that you not consider my role in Helena's recovery either as her luck or, even worse, as a mere coincidence that she found someone willing to stand by her. Personally, I take it as proof that everything can be achieved if you put enough energy into it, no matter what. I know what someone may say to all this. Such as: I am afraid, I do not have so much energy, and so on. It is in our human nature to find an excuse when something "big" needs to be done. Most often it is a fear of trying new things. To be honest, it was the same with us. But the situation had become so bad that we (or should I say Helena) had no other option than to start doing something about it. Does it sound familiar?

Domen Smole

Acknowledgements

My persistence in life is not just a matter of my innate character, my up-bringing also added to it. At this point I would like to thank my parents, Nataša and Milan, and my grandmother Jožefa for offering me a happy and most inspiring childhood. I would also like to thank my parents and my brother Andrej for being there for me in sickness and in health.

My thanks also go to my friend Michael, who visited me in the psychiatric clinic of Göttingen. Let me also thank my brother, my mother, Luka and his parents for "rescuing" me from the locked ward of the same clinic. Not that I didn't need to be locked up, but it felt great to get back home to Slovenia anyway.

Let me thank those of you who made it absolutely impossible for me to commit suicide in November 1996 — all my friends who came to visit: Nataša, Damjan, Tadeja, Andreja, Nina, Tina, Blaž, Igor, Leon, Špela, Barbara, and Katja.

Allow me thank all my friends who offered me a place to stay, helped me get medical help, and visited me in the psychiatric clinic of Ljubljana in October and November 1997. Thank you Aleš B., Andrej S., Janja, Tadeja, Andreja, Aleš R., and Mateja.

The last psychotic episode in 2003 was the first and hopefully the last my husband Domen had to put up with. It was a test of our relationship. I am glad he managed to find the strength to hang on and support me. I cannot find the words to thank him for all he did and is still doing for me. I would also like to thank his family: Breda, Jani, Katja, and Urška for accepting me the way I am and for not clinging to some boring stigmas. And last but not least, I would like to thank my friends who came to visit me at the psychiatric clinic of Ljubljana in 2003: Mojca, Andreja, Tadeja, and Hannah.

Thank you Ante for lending me the book by L. Hay You Can Heal Your Life in 2004. It changed my life.

In addition to my relatives and friends who stood by me at all times, I would also like to thank all the psychiatrists, psychotherapists, and alternative healers who helped me through the years. They appear in alphabetical order: Louise Hay, Klelija Hrovatič (MD, Psychiatrist), Leo Ivandič, Dr. Tsultrim Kalsang, Magdalena Kovač, Phyllis Krystal, Nina Leskovar, Suzana Oreški (PhD), Terezija Oven (MD – General Medicine Doctor), Lucijan Podkrajšek (MD, Psychiatrist), Viktor Pogačar, Emil Roglič, Janez Rugelj (MD, PhD, Psychiatrist), Franc Štrus (MD, PhD, Psychiatrist), Boštjan Trtnik, and others.

Finally, I would like to thank the peer-reviewers of this book. They appear in alphabetical order as well: Professor Mojca Zvezdana Dernovšek (MD, PhD, Psychiatrist), Lejla Doberšek (MD – General Medicine Doctor), Mojca Hrabar, Dr. Tsultrim Kalsang, Miha Kordiš, Peggy McColl, Alenka Helena Petek (MD, Psychiatrist), Professor Rok Tavčar (MD, PhD, Psychiatrist, Head of the Rehabilitation Department, Psychiatric Clinic of Ljubljana), Mirjana Zalar.

Disclaimer

The author of this book does not provide medical advice nor recommend the use of any technique as a form of treatment for physical, emotional, or medical problems without the advice of a physician – there is no such advice by the author of this book, neither directly written in this book nor implied indirectly therein. The intent of the author is only to offer information of a general nature to help readers in their quest for well-being. In the event you use any of the information in this book, which is your right, the author and the publisher assume no responsibility for your actions. This book is not a recipe, it is merely an inspiration.

Contents

1   **INTRODUCTION**

7   **CHAPTER ONE**
My Story
- *9*   The "luggage" I brought to Germany, where I fell ill
- *11*   October 1996, Göttingen, Germany:
  My First Schizoaffective Disorder (SchAD) Episode
- *17*   November 1996–June 1997:
  Writing My Final Thesis at Home
- *20*   October 1997, Graz, Austria:
  My Second SchAD Episode
- *24*   March 1998 – December 1998:
  Final Exams and Graduation
- *25*   November 1998:
  I Joined My First Alternative Therapy Group
- *27*   January 1999: My First Job
- *27*   October 1999: I Met My Future Husband
- *27*   October 2000: I Started Master's Degree Studies
- *29*   June 2003: I Attended My First Business Seminar
- *29*   October 2003: My Third SchAD Episode

31   **CHAPTER TWO**
Face it girl, you have schizoaffective disorder
- *33*   The Problem of Denial and Fear
- *35*   Dealing with Fear
- *38*   Positive Thinking for Mental Patients – Start Small

CHAPTER THREE
Waltz with your schizoaffective disorder – Learn to separate your personality from your SchAD

- 45   The Era of Indigo Children
- 50   Our Character and SchAD
- 54   The Possibility of Character Flaw Improvements
- 60   The Magical Power of our Effort

CHAPTER FOUR
Take the SchAD-bull by the horns – Identify your present fears and try to find their origin in your past in order to finally eliminate them

- 69   Warning
- 70   The Real You
- 72   An Example of Analyzing My Fears That Originate from My Past
- 76   Finding the Bright Side of Tragic Events

CHAPTER FIVE
Taming your schizoaffective disorder – Practical tips for people with a mental illness

- 83   The Big Picture
- 84   Why me?
- 86   We Should View Our Sensitive Brain as a Precious Jewel
- 87   Is schizoaffective disorder an illness of the soul or one of the body? My view of the dilemma
- 88   Fighting on Many Fronts: Western Medicine, Mental Exercises, Natural Healing, Lifestyle Choice
- 96   You have changed your way of thinking into a more positive one, but now you feel uncomfortable about it – what to do?

97	Choose the people you hang out with
100	The Importance of Listening to People Who Live with Us and Care about Us
102	When should you tell people about your mental illness?
104	Little Innocent Addictions of Every Day Life
105	Saying Thanks as a Habit
108	Keep your spirits up!
109	**EPILOGUE** **Failure is not an option. Says who?**
113	**MY DAILY ROUTINE**
119	**AN OVERVIEW OF ALL THE PERSONAL GROWTH SEMINARS I HAVE TAKEN PART IN**
123	**Glossary of Terms**
127	**Endnotes**
129	**Index**

INTRODUCTION

Why have I produced a light-hearted book about a very serious illness? I decided to write a book about my first-hand experience with mental illness in order to help other mental patients. I have written it from the heart. However, I also checked similar books on the market. I believe I managed to figure out what people most need in addition to the present array of books written by people like me. In my opinion, we might benefit from a bright approach, an optimistic story spiced with some humorous anecdotes. The most difficult things in life are easier if we manage to laugh about them.

Apart from what I believe could be viewed as the added value of this book, I also wanted to come "out of the closet". Many people have already spoken about their mental illness publicly. Nonetheless, in my opinion there could not possibly be too many of us speaking about our mental illnesses, for the dreaded stigma of mental illness is still present. As far as so-called de-stigmatization is concerned, I hereby claim to specialize in inner de-stigmatization. Let me rephrase it very simply: I believe that the stickiest and the most dangerous label on our foreheads are the labels we stick there ourselves. Thus this book is not so much oriented to the mentally healthy people who are told to accept us, as is recommended to my co-patients, who are told to accept themselves the way they are – their mental illness included. Please see Chapter Two regarding how to face the fact that you have a mental illness.

As far as such stigma is concerned, it is irrelevant what my precise diagnosis is. Thus I speak about mental illness in general in this respect. However, all other aspects of my mental illness are specific at least to some extent. Thus, I must emphasize already in this chapter that I have a schizoaffective disorder – bipolar type. I choose to abbreviate it SchAD.

If you read the first halves of the titles of Chapters Three to Five of this book they seem to tell a story:

- Waltz with your schizoaffective disorder. –
- Take the SchAD-bull by the horns. –
- Taming your schizoaffective disorder. –

First you dance with your disorder, meaning that you differentiate yourself from it: "I am not the schizoaffective disorder. SchAD is something I have". This step is very important, since there is always the danger that we assign also our personality traits to the disorder we have. For example, if we are very thoughtful and careful as a person, we might think that we are experiencing clinical anxiety in situations when we are worried about something real. In reality not every worry is a symptom of an illness. Sometimes we are worried about a real situation, but we think we have a symptom of anxiety.

In addition to that, there is another very common danger in identifying ourselves with the illness too strongly. We tend to become so immersed in our illness that we forget who we really are. We tend to see only the symptoms of our mental illness and we no longer notice our virtues. Such ways of thinking lead to low self-esteem.

Let me give you an example of how we can learn to view our symptoms of mental illness merely as biochemical irregularities in our brain: when I feel suicidal, I tell myself: "Oh, that is not me wanting to die. It is just that those biochemicals in my brain have become messed up again. They force me to feel suicidal. I do not really mean it."

After having successfully separated our personality from our disease, we can learn to live with it. First we "take the SchAD-bull by the horns", which means we analyze our past. In Chapter Four I give my personal example of how I managed to find the origins of my fear of doctors in my past, and have gradually gotten rid of it. I wish to warn readers about two things here. First, do not try to analyze your past without medical assistance. And second, remember that not every fear has an origin in your past. Some fears are merely biochemical irregularities in your brain.

"Taming your schizoaffective disorder" means learning to live with it as well. I have gathered together various practical tips in Chapter Five.

I wanted to make the chapter titles more colorful and motivational by adding some imagery in the first part of the title. The illustrations serve the same purpose. They are intended to make a very serious and painful illness a bit easier to bear.

My story is not a recipe for anyone else. You should consult your psychiatrist before trying any of the methods mentioned in this book. However, my story will hopefully encourage you to keep fighting for a healthy life. If I made it, so can you.

I quote several new age books in this book. My intention was to show that changing our thinking patterns really works. And even more importantly: that it works for mental patients too.

The stories told in this book are all true stories. All the names of the individuals involved have been left out to protect their privacy.

If you would like to read my blogs, you are welcome to visit my website at: **http://www.helenasmole.com** .

CHAPTER ONE

My story

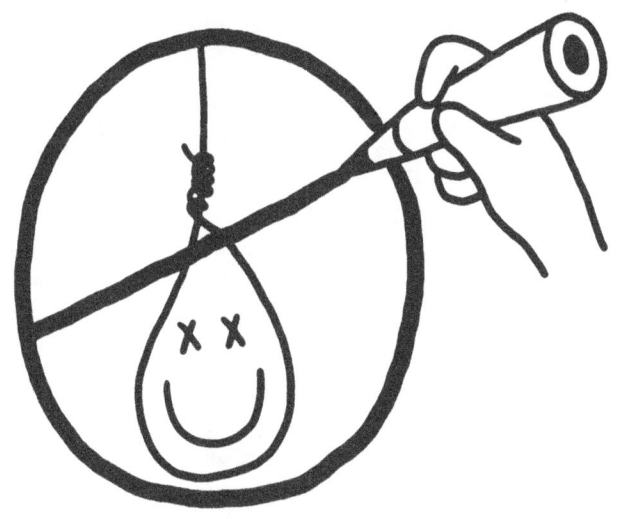

The "luggage" I brought to Germany, where I fell ill.

Let me give you a bit more information about my background first. I am Slovene. Slovenia used to be a part of ex-Yugoslavia, now it is an independent state and a part of the European Union. To put it more simply, we are a Slavic nation and live in an independent state situated between Italy, Austria, Hungary, and Croatia.

My story is actually a classic one. I was an 'A-student' that fell ill all of a sudden and nobody had a clue how this could have happened. It happened in a peculiar situation though.

At university I studied German language and literature as one "major" and journalism as a second "major". Back then a Bachelor of Arts study program lasted five years. We had lectures for four years. We had exams every half a year. At the end of the four years we had a year to write our final thesis. Our faculty also required the students to take overall final exams in this last year. Those were the most difficult exams. We had to memorize the whole history of German literature again. It was approximately one fifth of all the lectures we had listened to in the previous four years. Or in other words: we had to study the material for the regular exams we had already passed during the four years of lectures.

I started studying at the University of Ljubljana in the fall of 1992. After four years — in the fall of 1996 — I had only the final thesis left to write and the final exams to take. This was not very common. The majority of students had some of the regular semester-exams to catch up on before they could start writing their final thesis. I was happy to have accomplished that. I was also very happy to have been granted a scholarship to study at the University of Göttingen. From the psychiatric viewpoint, I believe I was **too happy** or better said, **abnormally happy**.

Thus I was really looking forward to spending five months in Germany. The scholarship was granted to me by DAAD (Deutscher Akademischer Austauschdienst – the German Organization for Academic Exchange). I went to Göttingen alone, so I could expose myself to German language to the fullest extent. I thought: "If I go somewhere where also some of my classmates are going, we will speak Slovene most of the time." What a mistake this turned out to be later, when I fell ill and had nobody to turn to.

Next to this "**abnormal joy**" there was another heavy bag amongst the luggage I took with me to Germany. It was the **pain** that had started already in the spring of 1996, which means about half a year prior going to Germany. I had not known how to deal with that pain. Thus I had just swallowed it and tried to bury myself in work in order to forget. Forget what? Forget the fact that my university-years boyfriend and I had broken up in February 1996. I had finished my semester exams by the end of the summer, but I had neglected my soul entirely. Thus the pain over the break-up was very much alive when I arrived in Göttingen in October 1996.

October 1996, Göttingen, Germany:
My First Schizoaffective Disorder (SchAD) Episode

I would like to share with you what my first schizoaffective disorder episode looked like. The description of a nightmare occurring in an awake state might scare readers that have never experienced anything like that. However, I am sure it will not be scary to those who have been psychotic before. Of course I have to tell you about the real situation as well. In order to make it easier for you to distinguish between the real world and my delusions, I have marked the delusions with *italics*. This holds only for this chapter of course. The italics in other chapters are not signs of any delusions. There is also another thing you have to know about this story. Back then in October 1996 I gradually started to lose track of time. So the beginning will sound logical and chronological. However, afterwards you will be thrown into a space-time continuum chaos, just like I was. I hope you do not mind ;-).

Drum roll please… here comes the psycho-thriller that took place in my head…

I started feeling weird right after my arrival in Göttingen. Two extreme moods were switching back and forth. The first one actually felt great. It was extreme joy and enormous self-confidence. *I felt I could move mountains. I remember joining a drama group and assuring the director I could memorize the major part in a fortnight.* He did not know how to react, for any sane people present knew that was impossible. Of course back then I was not aware that this state is referred to as **manic**. The other mood was horrible. *I was scared to death of making a mistake. And I also felt all alone. I needed company like a little* *baby needs his mother — all the time.* The fact that I was in a foreign country aggravated that feeling, even though I was starting to make new friends in Göttingen. However, back then I did not know this was a state of **depression** and **anxiety**.

I remember contacting my mentor, going to classes, meeting new people all the time. But most of all, I remember how I tried to sit behind the desk in my room in the student dormitory. I tried to do my homework but I could not. My **concentration** was so low, I did not know what I was reading. I also remember worrying a lot. *I was afraid there would be some penalty for not accomplishing what I had promised to accomplish.*

Let me explain. A year prior to my semester in Göttingen I had applied for a grant for financial aid during this semester. In the application for the grant we were supposed to present our study plans for the semester in Germany. These plans were not a promise though. And there was no penalty. However, I did not know back then that this *fear of a penalty* was already an early **paranoia**.

I can reconstruct what happened to some extent with the help of an insurance company document posted to Slovenia much later. I think this manic-depressive state must have lasted about 3 weeks. After that it got worse. *After this first phase of mental illness I completely lost track of time.* Parallel to losing track of time, I also started having **sleeping disorders** and I started **talking total nonsense** to my relatives in Slovenia on the phone.

As a result, my mother and brother drove by car about 600 miles to get to Göttingen and take me home. I rebelled and sent them back home, which for them meant another 600 miles in vain. *In my ill brain there grew the stupid idea that they were trying to take away from me what I had long been yearning for — a 5-month-stay in a German-speaking country and studying at a foreign university.* What a mistake to send them back. Things got really ugly after that. A full blown **psychosis** broke out.

The first sign that made me aware of the fact that something was wrong with my health was a sharp pain in my chest that would not go away. I tried to stay in the company of others at all times, but the students in the neighboring rooms could not talk to me day and night. I remember one early morning walking along our corridor in the student dormitory. In fact, walking is not the right word to describe what I was doing. *It was more like creeping in an upright position. I remember wanting to move along the corridor and find the door of a girl that seemed nice. Yet I could not read the names on the doors. It was like a real nightmare.* It is very difficult to describe what was going on in my head, but I remember the predominant feeling of *being trapped in a semi-awake state.*

It got worse. *I started believing and I had no doubt whatsoever that my ex-boyfriend had implanted a computer chip in my brain. He did this in order to help me forget him.*

How sweet of him, right? It is easy to joke about it now. However, back then these things were super scary.

I also believed that this "surveillance-system" was somehow connected to the heating radiator in my room. So I tried to stay out of my room as much as possible. Since I did not sleep much and I also was not really aware of the night and day sequence, I would wander around the city in the middle of the night.

I remember one night I put a coat on over my pajamas and went for a walk. *In the middle of the street I heard a phone ringing. The sound was as loud as if I were next to a phone.* And I did not possess a mobile phone back then. So I believe this was my first **hallucination**. I also remember that *at some point I did not know where I was any more.* But then there is a blank in my memory. I do not know how I got back to the student dormitory. The next thing I remember is waking up in my bed. I must have slept for a few hours. Then I went to see a doctor.

He asked me if there were some relatives in Germany he could phone. Of course there were none. He had no choice but to call an ambulance. I remember two very nice guys taking me to the ambulance. I remember telling them my life story and they seemed genuinely interested. I felt safe with them. It was soothing. But then – oh no – what a shock. The locked ward of the psychiatric clinic. Locked doors. What a shock. You can never explain to an ill person that such locks are good for them.

Life was not easy for me. There came another shock. The receptionist asked me: "Where are you from?" I said: "Slovenia." He answered: "Yes, sure." He did not believe me. Now this might seem like a hallucination, but it was not. The problem was that after a month in Germany having spoken only German, I started to speak German fluently. To him just a little misunderstanding – but to me this was a trigger of even more fear. Luckily I was sane enough to pull my passport out of my bag and resolve the mystery.

I do not remember much else from the clinic since I was sleeping most of the time due to the medication I was given. Luckily it calmed my brain down.

Much later I found out that I had spent 13 days locked in that clinic. This information was written on that insurance company document mentioned above. On the 12th day my mother and my ex-boyfriend arrived from Slovenia at the psychiatric clinic in Göttingen. This time I agreed to go home. However, I planned to be back in a fortnight. Of course I did not know it takes much longer to get well after a psychotic episode. And most importantly, I still was not ready to let the terrific opportunity of an academic exchange slip through my fingers.

My mother had come to Germany carrying a very important document, signed by the head of the psychiatric clinic of Ljubljana, Slovenia. He personally vouched for me, for I was in no condition to travel. Especially not by train. Luckily my ex-boyfriend's mother worked in another clinic in Slovenia, so she spoke to the head of the psychiatric clinic. In short, it was a rescue mission. Luckily again, I was insured. The hospitalization would have cost my parents a fortune.

So we drove home – my mother, my ex-boyfriend, and me – by train. Pretty soon I realized I was not going back to Germany in a fortnight. It was the end of the world for me. Not so much because of the failed foreign stay and studies, but because I was "officially nuts" at that point. I did not know the exact diagnosis, but I knew I was mentally ill. Back then psychiatrists would not tell you the exact diagnosis right at the beginning, for they thought it would only make you feel worse. I cannot speak for everyone, but if I may speak for myself – it was better this way. For I was not ready to accept my mental illness anyway.

Thus I found out what my official diagnosis was only years later: **schizoaffective disorder – bipolar type**. It happened by mistake. I was peeking in some official medical papers lying in front of me on the desk of my psychiatrist. At that point my psychiatrist explained to me what **schizoaffective disorder – bipolar type** means. I do not remember her exact explanation. You can look up more professional definitions on the internet, but let me give you a very simplified version here. For me schizoaffective disorder – bipolar type is a combination of **schizophrenia** and **bipolar disorder**. Bipolar disorder is called *bi*-polar, because it includes **both** manic and depressive symptoms. I have described both of them above. All the other symptoms I had (paranoia and other delusions, hallucinations) are typical of schizophrenia. I am well aware of the fact that a simple list of symptoms is not the definition of schizophrenia. However, it would be beyond the scope of this book to argue about the difference between schizophrenia and schizoaffective disorder.

Since I will be mentioning schizoaffective disorder a lot in this book, I have chosen to abbreviate it as follows: **SchAD**. Since SAD usually means seasonal affective disorder, I chose to abbreviate schizoaffective disorder in a slightly different way – SchAD. The abbreviation says nothing about the bipolar type – again it is beyond the scope of this book to talk about precise diagnosis classification. For those who would like to have the big picture of things presented anyway – let me tell you that there are two types of SchAD. There is the above mentioned bipolar type, and another one called depressive type. The second type lacks manic symptoms – that is the most important difference between the two types.

November 1996–June 1997:
Writing My Final Thesis at Home

When the doctors had stabilized my condition with medication in November 1996, I became aware of what had happened. I felt lost. The world as I knew it had crumbled in a month. I was very desperate. Thinking of suicide became my **new** and also **my only** "hobby".

There I was – back at my parents' house, feeling like a piece of sh**. Not that my parents are bad people – on the contrary. Nevertheless, in my opinion I was a little girl again. Or better put: I felt that my "brilliant career" had ended before even properly beginning. There I was, lying in bed all day with a concentration capacity close to zero. Me – a former A-student who could study in deep concentration for 8 hours a day. I am talking about the net amount – all breaks deducted. At that point in November 1996 I could not sit behind a desk for half a minute.

And I had to write my final thesis. How? Would somebody please tell me how? I had no answer. Nobody had said I should start writing the thesis in November of 1996. I was pushing myself because I had been used to working most of the time. And in that foggy November I was incapable of any work whatsoever. I felt as if I had hit a wall.

Today I am grateful for that wall, but back then it felt like the end of the world for me. By becoming single and by not being able to study, I lost everything. Or at least that was how I thought back then. I was somehow back to square one after all the effort I had put in studying. Or perhaps I should say that was the way I felt. Today – when I read about homeless people with schizoaffective disorder – I realize how little I had actually lost back then. Today I see November 1996 as a reset, as a terrific opportunity to re-think my goals and values. Of course, you must know that we are talking about a time-span of 14 years from the first psychotic episode to this realization today.

Let me sum up how the situation looked to me in November 1996 when I got back home. I had to start working on my final thesis, but I was not able to concentrate. I was convinced I would never have another love relationship, for guys "do not like girls who are officially nuts". I was getting fat due to the pills I was taking. I had no will power whatsoever. Pretty scary. *I felt trapped. As if life itself had put me in a straitjacket.* Until New Year I did not do much. *I could not even watch TV, since every movie scared me, even comedies. I totally misunderstood everything. I remember being scared of the TV character Alf, a friendly puppet.* Luckily the medication worked, so I slept normally and I did not hallucinate. I also did not have any paranoid stories going round in my head, like the one involving the implanted computer chip.

However, I was very worried about everything. So in January

1997 I persuaded my mother to go with me back to Göttingen. We went by train to pick up my dictionaries, clean my room, transfer the unspent money back to the academic exchange institution that had given me the scholarship, and to post some borrowed books to the students that had lent them to me. Of course the money could have been transferred from Slovenia, the students would have survived without those few paperbacks, and new dictionaries would have cost me less than the two train tickets. But O.K. – at least I did not start fantasizing about staying in Göttigen.

Two months after my arrival back home from Germany, the Slovenian psychiatrist that had taken over from where the German psychiatrists successfully started, said: "You are relatively stable now. Maybe you could try to work on your thesis. Little by little."

It was easier said than done, but I put myself to work. The first days I could only sit at the table and study for about three minutes. It looked hopeless. Yet I would not give up. I was adding to my minutes over the weeks and sometime around Easter I was done. I had read through all the material and I had underlined all the relevant sentences. Work that would normally have taken me a month had taken me three months. Of course in the first month I accomplished almost nothing. Due to my perseverance and the medication I was able to do most of the research for my final thesis in the last month before Easter.

Now, when I look back on this, I do not feel sorry for myself. On the contrary – my destiny gave me a great opportunity to prove I CAN "move some lower mountains", if I decide to do so. And I finally understood children and teenagers who cannot study due to a lack of concentration.

Writing my final thesis after having read all the material was easy. It took me only a fortnight. I even came up with an original idea to be added to the quoted findings. I was starting to feel better. The thesis was approved. There was no bachelor's degree thesis defense back then. Students had to take three final exams instead. As mentioned above, those three exams were the most difficult ones of the whole Bachelor of Arts program. They were difficult because it was impossible to memorize all the facts we were required to know by heart. Even to memorize half of the facts took a lot of time, effort, and willpower.

However, instead of preparing for those three exams, I chose to go to Austria for a semester. I was not willing to give up my strong desire to spend a semester in a German speaking country. Then came my next mistake. This time it was closer to my home. I chose Graz, a city in Austria. It was only about 180 miles away from my home. Nonetheless, I should not have left home.

October 1997, Graz, Austria: My Second SchAD Episode

I decided to give it another shot. I applied for a scholarship for a semester at the University of Graz granted by ÖAD (Österreichischer Akademischer Austauschdienst – the Austrian Organization for Academic Exchange) in February

1997. My mother thought it was not a good idea. Nevertheless, I persisted in making my big dream happen. I desperately wanted to spend a semester studying in a German-speaking country. It had been my plan for years. I did not want to abandon this plan. I wanted to give it another try. I thought: "If I can make this plan happen, my psychiatric past will be over and done, completely forgotten. There will be no more stigma." The scholarship was approved in early summer 1997. I was granted a scholarship for a semester in Graz, starting in October 1997, a year after my first SchAD episode. Of course I did not tell my psychiatrist about my plans.

In June 1997 I told my psychiatrist my final thesis was finished. I was stabilized. He said it was possible that I had only had one psychotic episode and that would be it. Since I had responded to the medication so well and finished my final thesis, he proposed that I take a chance and try being without medication. I agreed instantly with enthusiasm. Of course, he explicitly told me to start taking the pills again the very moment I noticed anything strange.

I was rather happy. Still a bit "biochemically depressed" after the first SchAD episode, but rather happy. It seemed everything was going to be all right at that moment. I was off pills, which for me meant that I was officially NOT a psychiatric patient anymore. The label of psychiatric patient was probably even more troublesome than the past symptoms of the mental illness I had been through. I was declared cured, or in my terms "not-officially-nuts anymore". That was it for me. A load off of my shoulders.

So in October 1997 my brother took me to Graz by car. I was not aware of it back then, but I was a bit manic already before leaving my home country. In Graz deep depression set in, which was occasionally interrupted by manic behavior. I had difficulty falling asleep in the evenings. I think I had been less than a fortnight abroad when my second psychotic episode occurred. *First I had some weird flashbacks that seemed like a movie about my life. Everything seemed to make sense, although as far as can I remember, the sense itself was somewhat weird.* I do not remember the story of the flashbacks anymore. At that moment I was still able to get some hours of sleep at night. Only it got worse with time. *I became convinced that the students in the student dormitory where I lived were putting poison in my food.* We had a common refrigerator for the whole floor, *so there it was – waiting for them to poison it.* I remember one night weeping all night long. My roommate begged me to take my medication. I refused. I was not ready to put the label on my forehead again. For in my opinion that was what taking antipsychotic medication meant. What I thought to myself back then was pretty simple: "If I take medication, I am nuts. If I manage to survive without medication, I am sane." This kind of thinking was pretty stupid of course, for in reality it is the other way around.

However, despite my full-blown SchAD episode I must have had some sense of the people around me. I was aware of the fact that I was disturbing my roommate, so I decided to go back to Slovenia.

The trip back home was a psychotic experience. I remember taking enough cash for the train ticket and leaving the room. I started to walk towards the train station, which was about an hour away from the student dormitory on foot. I could have taken the bus, but I felt a strong urge to walk, for I had too much energy. A lot of things happened on the way to the train station. First I saw a postcard in front of a shop. The postcard pictured a cute little witch. On top of the illustration there was a sentence: "I am a witch." My first thought was: *"They have put this postcard here to make me realize I am a witch. It is not a coincidence. I am a witch. Right! That explains everything. That is why I can read people's minds."* In short – I had **megalomaniacal ideas**.

Afterwards I remember buying all kinds of things. Before arriving at the train station I had spent all the cash I had taken with me. So I had to go back to my room in the student dormitory to pick up some more money. And then again I went on foot towards the train station. It must have taken me half a day to eventually get to the train station with some actual money for the train ticket. At the train station I waited for quite a long time, for I had not planned in advance which train I would catch. I remember observing three ladies. *I was absolutely certain they were three witches of good will. I thought they were watching over me. They made me feel safe.*

The train took me to Ljubljana. I did not want to go further west to my parents. It would have made me feel like a little girl that had made the same mistake again. I was too proud to admit that.

In Ljubljana I lost track of time, but I will try to describe it chronologically anyway. I contacted various friends there.

They offered me a place to stay. *First I agreed, but then I got scared and disappeared.* I phoned the last friend in the middle of the night, after having wandered around the city. She picked me up and took me to her friend who was studying medicine back then. *I kept saying I was poisoned. I even carried a sample of my urine with me to be able to prove it. I thought the poison was some kind of illegal drug.* The guy who studied medicine looked at my retinas and decided to take me to the Ljubljana psychiatric clinic, for my retinas showed no sign of any drugs. The next day he and my friend drove to my parents to tell them I had been hospitalized.

I stayed in the clinic for 2 months. One would think that would teach me a lesson. It did not. After being released from the psychiatric clinic, I took a train back to Graz. Due to the medication I was functioning normally. However, I was not able to concentrate while reading. I attended some lectures and tried to make some notes. I am sure they were not any good. I took a train back to Slovenia every fortnight for a check up at my psychiatrist's. I returned right after each check up. Today, when I look back, this was very stupid. I should have stayed home, since I was not able to study anyway.

March 1998 – December 1998: Final Exams and Graduation

In spring 1998 I still had my final exams at the University of Ljubljana to finish. Again my concentration was poor. Yet I did it. I finished all three exams by December 1998. A friend of mine said: "You finished your bachelor's degree only because you are as stubborn as hell." I took it as a compliment. My stubbornness caused me to make a lot of mistakes. Yet it saw me through the marathon preparation for the three final exams as well.

During these months of preparation for the final exams I once joined a group of people that were competing in an orienteering race. I thought it would be doable for me too. And it would have been doable, had I not been too ambitious. At first the path looked rather level so I started running. After a few minutes of running I was faced with a hill. My running soon turned to very slow walking. It felt as if the hill had no peak while ascending. I somehow managed to reach the peak in the end. I was almost without energy at the top. And this was only the first short part of the whole route. I kept dragging myself towards the end of the route. I regretted having joined the competition. As a group we finished last because of me.

That hill at the beginning of the path became a metaphor for depression to me. You fight and fight and there is no way out. Well at least it seemed that way for quite some time. I remember that hill very well. The feeling of powerlessness that overwhelmed me going uphill was sharp and it has stayed in my memory until today.

November 1998:
I Joined My First Alternative Therapy Group
A month before graduation I joined a program for people with various psychological problems. The program was led by a

psychiatrist and psychotherapist who believed that one can do more about one's mental illness than just take medication. We had to do mountain hiking, marathon running, a lot of book reading, and even more writing about how we felt and what we thought about ourselves and the world around us. We were divided into groups. Each group met once a week for group talk therapy. Once a month there was a meeting of all the groups. I stayed in the program for two years.

This program helped me re-build my self-esteem, because I participated in running races. It also kept me in good physical shape. Back then I thought that entering a running race was nothing special. However, now that my self-image has improved, I am proud of myself for having run a marathon – 26 miles and 385 yards. I was the last, but I did it. In the talk therapy group sessions I learned a lot about relationships, for there were many couples attending the program for couple therapy.

At this point I would like to thank my brother, who accompanied me as a supportive partner in this psychotherapy and lifestyle change program. In order to help me he had to participate in all the mentioned activities. He really sacrificed a lot of time and energy for me. I would also like to thank my mother, who joined the program the last half year to support me.

January 1999:
My First Job

Two months after graduation I got my first and thus far only job. I was employed there for nine years. I quit in November 2008. I will analyze the causes of my decision to leave this job in Chapters Three, Four, and Five.

October 1999:
I Met My Future Husband

I met my future husband while running a 13-mile half marathon in October 1999. He was running in front of me. I sped up. I do not know what drove me to speed up at that point. I did not even see his face. It must have been destiny itself. After I had managed to run even with him, I started chatting with him. I looked at his face. He looked cute. Chatting with him made me feel safe, for I noticed very quickly that he was and still is very wise, thoughtful, and calm. Towards the end of my 13 miles I was running out of strength. I only made it because he was supporting me emotionally. He then ran another 13-mile circuit to complete the full 26-mile marathon. I waited for him at the end of the race carrying a warm blanket and a cup of hot tea. It was love at first sight.

October 2000:
I Started Master's Degree Studies

In October 2000 I decided to start master's degree studies in addition to my regular job. I could not do all three things at the same time, so I left the program for people with psychological problems described above. Yet I did not abandon all the new activities I had learned there. I still go mountain hiking or for easy nature walks. I had to stop running in 2001 due to a knee problem, but I started doing martial arts (ju-jitsu) the same year and continued for two years. Later I resumed running, but I never ran more than 5 miles, since the knee problem always reappeared when I tried to prolong the distance. In the last three years I have switched to oriental dance, which I find most appropriate for my body constitution and my psychological nature. I have also been doing the five Tibetan rejuvenating exercises in the morning for nearly six years.

As far as books are concerned, I still read a lot, as I always have. And as far as talk therapy is concerned, my husband and I talk everything through.

Since gaining my master's degree in 2005, I have attended various psychotherapy seminars, for I recognized the importance of doing more than just taking medication in the above mentioned Alternative Therapy Group already. You can find a complete list of all the seminars I have attended at the back of the book.

I entered a master's degree program in 2000 because I thought: "Maybe if I go into more depth regarding the knowledge my job requires, I will start enjoying it." It did not work, for my job was not what I was meant for in the first place. Writing this book is the first step on the path to fulfilling my real vocation. My mission in life is to make mental illness casual. In such a way we – mental patients – can remove the stigma we choose to carry by ourselves.

June 2003:
I Attended My First Business Seminar

Back in 2003 I attended my first business seminar ever. The first lecturer talked about the basic motivation to start one's own business. Or in other words: How to start doing something we really like before even thinking about the "big money" ahead. Back then I was not in the slightest ready to start my own business, but I remember two things the lecturer said:

1. She mentioned that negative thoughts were like weeds. If we want our plants (positive thoughts) to grow, we need to keep removing the weeds. Up until that moment I had thought that happy people did not have any negative thoughts at all. Wrong! We all have them. Happy people are just better gardeners.
2. She emphasized how important it was to find out WHAT WE REALLY LIKE DOING. She asked: "Do you ever jump up and down in the morning, because you are so happy to go to work?"

I could not relate to that jumping scene at all. I thought she was speaking science fiction. But she planted a seed in my head. A tricky question that kept popping up every time I felt dissatisfied with my job.

October 2003:
My Third SchAD Episode

Back then, in June 2003, the lecturer at that business seminar was one of the stars shimmering on the horizon. One of the stars that made it impossible for me to give up totally, no matter how depressed I felt. Yet I needed another psychotic episode later that year to force me to think.

My last SchAD outburst in 2003 was a classic manic-depressive cycle with a full-blown psychotic episode at the end. I stopped sleeping. *I had a paranoid theory of how some secret organization that was trying to prevent suicide was following me. I believed my phone was tapped and that there was even a listening device in my husband's car. When I was walking around I believed that the secret organization's representatives were also following me all over the city. It frightened me, but sometimes it also made me strangely secure. As far as megalomaniacal ideas are concerned, I thought I was the next Jesus Christ, taking all the suffering upon my shoulders. The hallucinations were not that bad, but still frightening. The colors of people's clothes in the streets seemed brighter than usual. I also believed that some friends of mine had been giving me poison in the form of chocolate. That poison, I believed, had caused the episode in the first place.*

I ended up in the locked ward of a psychiatric clinic. Again.

CHAPTER TWO

Face it girl,
you have schizoaffective disorder

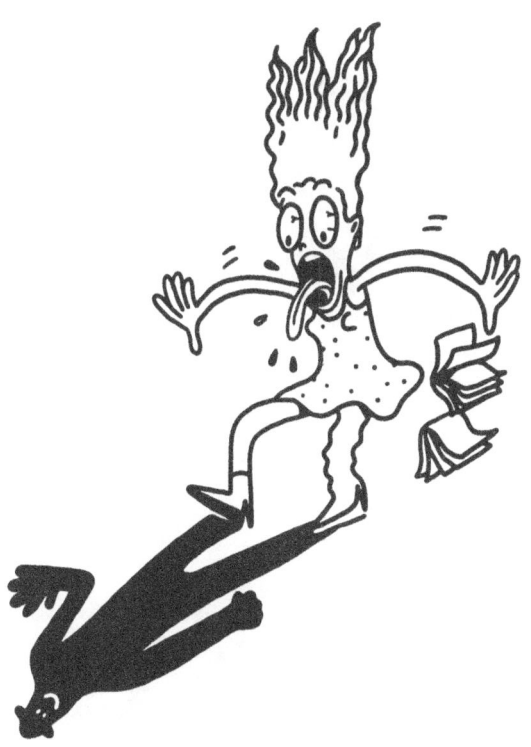

The Problem of Denial and Fear

When my first SchAD episode occurred, I did not want to accept the fact that I have a mental illness. I was ashamed that I had had to be locked in a psychiatric clinic. I was in denial. I stayed in denial for a very long time. Actually I do not know precisely when I finally accepted the fact that I have SchAD. Probably it was no sooner than in 2007, which means 11 years of denial. In April 2007 there was too much stress at work, so I experienced sleeping disorders. I remember listening to my future husband and thus seeing my psychiatrist soon enough to prevent a fourth SchAD episode. Maybe this could be observed as the full acceptance of my mental illness. Or maybe this book represents the ultimate acceptance, which sums up 14 years of denial. How is it possible that I was so stubborn?

Let me go back to November 1996, the time of my first SchAD episode. It felt horrible to have all those delusions and hallucinations. However, when I got stabilized with medication and was able to think normally, it felt just as horrible to face the facts. Not being able to study was tough, but accepting my diagnosis was even more difficult. Or shall I say – impossible. As mentioned above, I did not know my exact diagnosis back then, but I knew it must have been a serious mental illness, for I had hallucinated and had had paranoid thoughts. My first reaction was typical: "I do not have any mental illness. That is nonsense. I was just very stressed out. I should never have gone abroad so soon after a breakup with a boyfriend."

This denial went on for years and has taken on different forms. The first form was a wish to escape. I was trying desperately to make everything function as it had functioned before. And of course my mental illness episode was to remain top secret. However, the news spread, which terrified me. I thought to myself: "If people find out that I have been locked up in a psychiatric clinic, I will never get a boyfriend or a job."

Being terrified was the core emotion, the core way of my thinking. Fear was my whole new identity. And I remained immersed in fear for years. Me, once a rather brave person, totally tied up with ropes of fear. Gradually I forgot how it feels not to be scared all the time. My fear seemed to be the very driving force of the denial.

I worried constantly and worry by definition is fear of the future. There was always at least one catastrophic scenario to be afraid of at all times. The only way I could forget a scenario like this was to come up with another one. I was addicted to catastrophic scenarios.

I also acquired new **situational fears** I had not had before my first SchAD episode. I became afraid of traveling abroad, of being caught by darkness while walking in the mountains, of destroying a computer file by mistake, etc. The fear of traveling abroad might seem irrelevant to people living in a huge country like the USA, for example. But for a Slovene person, foreign countries are very close and almost indispensable as regards studying, business, or holiday trips. The highway that traverses the whole country of Slovenia is less than 200 miles long. Thus for a Slovene person, fear of traveling abroad is pretty claustrophobic.

Dealing with Fear

During my third episode I was hospitalized, as mentioned above. I was released from the psychiatric clinic just before Christmas 2003. In January 2004 I still had some energy left. I remember jogging around the complex of apartment buildings where I lived. I became very tired after a few minutes of running, though. So I walked the rest of the way. Still, I managed to keep up the routine of this morning exercise for a whole month. In February 2004 the so-called post-psychotic emptiness phase started. It was my worst depressive emptiness ever. I did nothing else but lie in bed day and night for two months. Then I persuaded my psychiatrist to end my sick leave, so that I would at least get up in the morning. I started to work 20 hours per week in April 2004.

However, I still lay in bed most of the time while at home. I hit rock bottom. I wanted to die. I had to do something. A friend of my husband's lent me a book by L. Hay, *You Can Heal Your Life*[1]. He also directed me to an alternative, bio-energy healer. She advised me to do the mental work described in this book. She was also the reason why I started to do the five Tibetan rejuvenating exercises every morning[2]. I have been doing them for six years now.

I started the mental work described in L. Hay's books in late spring 2004. I also knew already in 2004 that it was crucial for me to find out **what I really want to do for a living**. Yet I was only able to find that out in 2007.

Today I really feel that writing self-help books is what I want to do for a living. And it makes me happy. Had I not had that psychotic episode in 2003, I would probably still be clinging to my job and would remain semi-miserable for the rest of my life.

The book *You Can Heal Your Life* was another starting point in my efforts to improve my mental health in addition to taking prescribed medication. **The imagery or the so-called visualizations** and **mirror work or the so-called affirmations** described in this book were my first "mental exercises". I started to do them in the spring of 2004. The medication made me sleep at night and work in the daytime, which is very important in general and also indispensable as the basis for any mental work. However, I felt that if I wanted to be really happy, I would have to do more than just take the prescribed pills. A visualization exercise I picked up from Hay's book was, for example, the "little child exercise"[3]. You close your eyes and imagine yourself as a little child aged five or six. Then you look deeply into this little child's eyes. You reach out your arms and embrace this child, etc. This exercise helps you on the path towards loving and fully accepting yourself the way you are. The same goes for the so-called affirmations or mirror work described in the same book. You stand in front of the mirror, look yourself in the eye, and say out loud: "I love and appreciate myself". This sentence is just an example. You can find other suggestions and guidelines for creating your own sentences in the above mentioned book.

Along with Hay's recommended exercises, I remember doing another exercise suggested by my future husband. As mentioned above, I felt scared all the time, nonetheless once or twice a week I acquired an additional catastrophic scenario to be super-scared of. Those were the moments when I panicked. My future husband told me to ask myself the following question whenever I panicked: "What is the worst thing that can happen, if ...this and that... happens?" For example: "What is the worst thing that can happen if you destroy a computer file by mistake?" My answer would be: "I get fired." My husband's comment would be: "So you find another job." Of course I argued that I would never find another job, but my husband was really very patient with me and kept assuring me that none of my catastrophic scenarios led to the end of the world. We would talk for hours. Sometimes he managed to calm me down from the panic degree of fear to the usual degree of fear that was constant in those years (1996 – ca. 2006). Sometimes, however, even such conversations did not help much. Nonetheless, if I look at those talks with him from the point of view of today, I can say that gradually the question "What is the worst thing that can happen, if ...this and that... happens?" became more and more powerful. Gradually we came to the point where the answers to this question were able to calm me down and there was no further discussion. Of course this was no earlier than in 2007 or maybe in 2008.

I would like to stress here that I would never have made it without my husband supporting me at all times. This "fear exercise" is only a small part of our talks in the years described in this book. My husband's common sense was really therapeutic. So was his love for me. They both still **are** very therapeutic. I am a lucky girl indeed.

Positive Thinking for Mental Patients – Start Small

It took me 14 years starting with my first SchAD episode to be able to speak about my schizoaffective disorder publicly. It also took me 14 years to finally be able to see the bright side of it all.

Since no one can expect you to see the positive side of a mental illness right away, I would suggest something else. You should start with little things that happen to you in everyday life. Let me give you an example from my experience.

I was taking a walk when out of the blue there came a huge dog that wanted to meet me and leave some saliva on my coat. I am not a dog lover and I especially hate it if they lick my hands or clothes. So I took my coat to the dry cleaner's the next day. At first I thought to myself: "Damn dog. It cost me money!" But then I thought: "There must be something good about it. Let's wait. It may reveal itself later".

And it did! At the dry cleaner's they removed some thread balls that had become embedded in the back of the coat. I had been certain they could not be removed. The lady at the dry cleaner's managed to do so and I was surprised. The cleaning cost 12 euros, but the new coat I was planning to buy some time soon – for I thought the "thread balls" could not be gotten rid of – would have cost me 200 euros. So the dog actually saved me 188 Euros!

It is not easy to accept your SchAD just the way it is, for it is a nasty illness. So I suggest you start with an easier task. Why don't you first try to accept the way you look, for example? Let me tell you my story of gradually accepting myself the way I am.

In 2004 I started doing the mirror exercises described in the Hay's book mentioned above. I kept telling myself loudly while looking into the mirror: "I love and appreciate myself." It seemed weird at the beginning. I did not believe what I was saying. I was repeating it mechanically. However, when it did start to feel a bit real, I suddenly felt beautiful. I started to love the way I look. Then I kept repeating the sentence: "I love and appreciate myself." In time I began to love my personality. Needless to say my SchAD was the last thing about myself that I started to accept. And it took me five years of mirror exercises and other mental exercises to start loving myself just the way I am – my SchAD included. These days I still repeat: "I love and appreciate myself", whenever I feel sad or insecure. Mirror exercises have become a habit. So have some other mental exercises I write about in the following chapters.

Let me say something more about the way I look. I kept losing weight from puberty to 2007. I lost about 20 pounds four times and I always gained them back sooner or later. I took the hard path – I exercised and ate a lot of vegetables. I was losing 2 pounds per month. This is the sure way to lose weight. Well it did not work for me. I have always gained the 20 pounds back sooner or later. Usually I gained them in the last phase of a schizoaffective disorder episode, which in my case was always a depression spent predominantly in bed.

Then one day in 2007, after I had put on 20 pounds again, I said to myself: "I always gain back the 20 pounds. I never gain 30 pounds, for example. So what if 154 pounds is my ideal weight?" The moment I accepted the combination of my 154-pound weight at my height of 5 feet 5 inches as my "perfect body mass index" – I suddenly started to feel slim. It took me years of mental training to come to this realization described above. By the way, my body mass index (BMI) is 26, which is slightly overweight, but it is nothing serious.

I am not saying that a person who's BMI indicates obesity should just accept him- or herself the way they are and not lose any weight. On the contrary – they **should** lose weight. But they should also try to learn how to love him- or herself at the same time. This seems like a contradiction at first: "How am I supposed to lose weight, if I love myself the way I am. I should hate myself first, only then can I lose weight." However, the mathematics of this self-image formula is a bit more complicated than this.

In reality, true love gets into every fat cell – even if there are too many of them. The more you love yourself, the more time you reserve for yourself over the course of the day. In that special time reserved only for yourself you can do mental training, physical exercise, and you can carefully pick the food you eat. You will also be able to cook healthy food.

The common excuse for not being able to try this would be: "But I cannot reserve time just for myself. Others need me." Think! It might be the other way around. You might need the people around you to make you happy. And as they fail to do so, you want them even more to make you happy. It is a vicious circle. For the love you really seek comes from within you. When you accept yourself, you start loving yourself and you do not need other people so desperately anymore. When they start to feel that you are not clinging to them so much, they will love you even more. For you have set them free. It is a circle again, only this time it is a happy one, and no longer vicious.

In addition to your weight, make-up is also an important issue. I have learned not to "cover my spots" or "hide my flaws" anymore. I apply make-up on my face with totally different thoughts in mind. I concentrate on highlighting my virtues. It is a whole new perspective. Using the very same lipstick and eye-shadow you can add so much more to the way you look by loving yourself just the way you are. For the joy in your heart emanates through your skin.

CHAPTER THREE

Waltz with your schizoaffective disorder – Learn to separate your personality from your SchAD

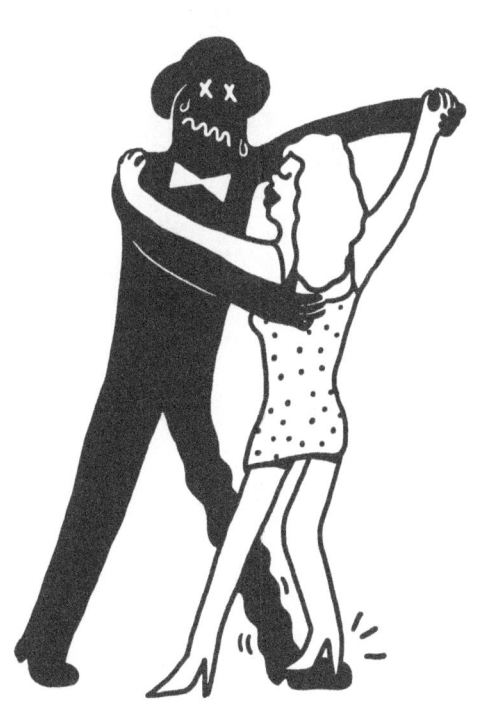

The Era of Indigo Children

The one personality trait that can easily be mistaken for a mental illness symptom is our indigo-children nature[4]. I am sure some of you have already heard about the so-called **indigo children phenomenon**, but let me explain in short what it means for those who have not. In the early 1970s clairvoyant people began to notice that a lot of children had an aura (the bio-magnetic field surrounding our bodies) of indigo color. This wave of "new children" still continues. These children are really special for they are somehow programmed to re-establish our ethical values by being very critical towards the school system and all other hierarchical state systems that lack integrity. In addition to that, indigo children, and some of them today already indigo adults, cannot conform to dysfunctional situations at home, work, or school. The indigos can sense dishonesty very quickly and cannot pretend everything is fine. Like I said, this kind of child is still being born, only after the turn of the millennium their aura has changed to a more opalescent color and therefore children born after 2000 are called crystal children. Crystal children are more even-tempered than the indigos, but they represent the same phenomenon.

As mentioned above, the early indigo children are today indigo adults and I think I am one of them too. However, it is not important whether you were born an indigo or not, for eventually everyone is becoming more like the indigo people. We are talking about a change in thinking of the whole human kind. This change is the mission of the indigo children and adults.

I choose to believe that the indigo children phenomenon is true despite the doubts of the official psychological and sociological perspective. It is interesting, though, that official science has noticed some changes too, for they talk about new generations: generation X and generation Y. Let me tell you how I see this issue from my perspective.

The first indigo children were supposedly born about a century ago. They were pioneers and pathbreakers. In the early 1970s, however, their numbers started to grow[5]. I am referring to the first wave of indigo children in the 70s. Thus some of them – or shall I say us – are in our late 30s now. We often present a challenge to our parents and also to our employers. As employees, we need to know two things:

1. Why does it make sense to do a certain job?
   How is it going to contribute to the strategy
   and goals of the whole company we work for?
   We need to see the big picture. It has to
   make sense. And the sense has to be honest.
2. And on the other hand, we also need to know:
   Why does it make sense to avoid certain
   actions? Again, it is the big picture and
   integrity that count.

We do not simply **obey orders**. We need explanations **why**. So please – all employers and parents: start thinking. We will not change. We were programmed to seek the meaning of life and our mission in life. You will not be able to stop us. We are here to help you rethink your visions, plans, procedures, and values. You are welcome to join the flow of our generation. It is a whole new era we are talking about. And thank you – all parents and employers – who have already recognized and accepted us – the indigos.

Let me give you an example of a conflict arising from my indigo nature. When I first started working at my former job in 1999, they gave me a very complicated text to type into the computer. I asked: "Why do I have to do it this way? What about scanning it?" They told me the process of converting scans into text files would take too much time. I understood and was OK with it. Still, it took me a year to type all 500 pages and in this time another question kept popping up: "What are we going to need this text for?" I never got any sensible answer. Still I kept typing, because I needed my salary.

Today I see why it was so difficult to persuade myself every morning to enter my office and start typing.

I had to keep telling myself every day: "You need the money. You are earning a decent salary by typing this text. You have no choice. You are a patient with a schizoaffective disorder. No one else is going to offer you a job. So…you cannot quit." But somehow none of these sentences made me really tranquil. They kept me working, but I daydreamed of quitting this job every day. Today I know why: I was not told what they were going to do with this text. Their vague answers never satisfied me.

I am not trying to blame anyone here. Later I realized they could not have told me why, for there was a constant conflict between two other colleagues in the team that made the whole future plans vague.

Some years later I felt personally entangled in the above

mentioned conflict, although I was not able to describe how. I was not physically entangled. Everyone outside my place of work kept telling me that the conflict between my colleagues at work **was not my problem**. But somehow I felt it **was** my problem too. **Today I know why**: The conflict in the team was constantly making our future plans vague. There was no certainty and thus no sense in working. At least not for a person like me, for my boss could not have told me **why**. At least not in a way I would have found satisfying. "We have to give you some work." is no answer for people like me. We have to see the big picture. **And if there is no big picture, our job does not make sense.**

There was something else that aggravated my despair at that time. I was given a 2000-page text to type into the computer. I asked my boss if I could at least **try** scanning the 2000 pages instead of typing them. My boss replied: "But if the computer does all the work, what will you be doing?" I exclaimed: "I am going to do research. I am a researcher!" My boss answered: "You are not qualified to do research. You have to finish your masters degree first." Of course I was allowed to do research in my spare time, so you can imagine how absurd those explanations sounded.

That combined with the ongoing conflict between two other colleagues in the team was simply too much for me to bear. In October 2003 I got the usual SchAD symptoms, but I was in denial. Thus I refused to take my medication. Subsequently, it got so bad that I ended up in a psychiatric clinic. I also gave notice just before going to the clinic, but I later revoked it, for the doctors in the clinic persuaded me to do so.

I am sure all the people in this story meant no harm. They were all trying to take care of me. But none of them understood the logic of an indigo child. For them I was a spoiled brat. They were talking about "delayed growing up".

On the other hand, this was my last stay in a psychiatric clinic. And there was also a bright side to it – the last SchAD episode finally made me read the book by L. Hay[6], already mentioned several times in this text. After some months of wallowing in self-pity, I started reading the book in the spring of 2004. The book saved my life.

A friend of mine had told me about the book already in 1997. I borrowed it from a local library, read some pages. However, as soon as I read that L. Hay was a cancer survivor, I thought to myself: "This book is for cancer patients, not for me." Then I returned the book to the library. I was not ready for the book's wisdom back then. Seven years later – after the last SchAD episode – a friend of my future husband's lent me the same book. I read the whole book over and over. I was only ready to read the book so many years later. **I had to hit rock bottom first!**

Many times in my life I have been told: "You are stupid to be so honest." Back then I had my second thoughts, but the only things I regret today are my dishonest words and deeds. After I had read a book by P. McColl[7], which explains that we cannot be too honest, I felt relieved. It does not mean that I never make mistakes. It means that I **believe** in honesty. I used to hate myself for being honest, now I love myself whenever I manage to act, speak, or think honestly. Now that I have read how indigo children have a radar for dishonesty and that they cannot tolerate it, I know that I am on the right track again. These new children are said to have been sent to this planet in order to transform our way of thinking and that we should join them regardless of the fact whether we were born as indigos or not[8].

To sum up, it is crucial to accept the fact that we as humanity are moving to a new era. The child and adult indigos are showing the way. I think I am an indigo adult too, and that has nothing to do with my SchAD. I find it very important to separate these two things: my indigo nature and my mental illness. For if I put everything in the same basket, pretty soon I would start thinking I am nothing **but** my SchAD.

Our Character and SchAD

When SchAD first strikes it is very hard to discern our **mental illness** from our **innate character**. For example, we might think we are fearful. In fact, we might be brave as a person, but we experience anxiety as a symptom of our mental illness. It is the brain that has been exposed to too much stress and starts to act weird as a consequence of stress. If our brain is the most sensitive organ in our body, then it is precisely the brain that will fall ill in times of stress. So my suggestion would be: **Let us explore our character in times when we are healthy.** That way we will be able to see future episodes as merely a **mental illness that has nothing to do with our character**. That way we will help improve our self-image, which so easily gets destroyed already by the first mental illness episode. To be more concrete: we are still strong as a person, it is just the biochemicals in our brain that produce anxiety. Hereby I mean the natural substances in our brain, such as dopamine. To put it very simply, they are the molecules responsible for communication between nerve cells in the brain. Some mental illness symptoms are then due to irregular levels of dopamine, for instance.

Of course it might also be the other way around. We might see a character flaw that we have always had as a symptom of a mental illness that has just occurred. Again I would suggest: **Let us explore our character in times when we are healthy.** Thus we will be able to discern **our flaws of character that have absolutely nothing to do with our mental illness**.

Let me give you an example. First I will tell you a story from my past. Then I will try to depict my character flaws from the story.

The Story. I had been giving German lessons to a high school student for half a year. First he kept getting good grades in German and I was proud to be doing a good job. Then all of a sudden he got a failing mark. I panicked. What had I done wrong?

I phoned his mother and asked her: "How did it happen?" I reacted as if it were the end of the world. She explained that the teacher had come into the classroom five minutes late. After half an hour she wanted to collect the papers of all the pupils, although only a few were cheating. This would have left the students with only 30 minutes to complete the tasks instead of the usual 45 minutes. My student thought it was unfair, so he burst out in anger and insisted that the teacher does not collect the papers. He was successful, but I can imagine he only helped his colleagues. He, on the other hand, lost his concentration due to his outburst. As an addendum to this story, I was aware of the fact that my pupil had had a flue just before the test, so he was not even able to thoroughly prepare for the test.

Nonetheless, all these facts pointing in directions other than mine did not satisfy me. I still felt guilty. Afterwards I managed to come up with four improvements to my pedagogical methods and wrote them down. I felt a bit better. The next day my pupil came over for another private lesson. When I presented the new methods, he got upset, for the methods meant that he would have to work harder.

"There is nothing to worry about. I have gotten many failing grades before, but I have always managed to finish the school year with a satisfactory grade", he exclaimed. Two worlds crashed there: the world of a formerly diligent student and the world of a more easygoing, current high school student.

I kept picturing the line in my mind that our teacher at the school for emotional intelligence I was attending that year kept drawing on the table. It was the line between ME and YOU in a relationship. The line is supposed to remind us that we can only take care of 50% of the relationship. Yet somehow I was not completely calm about that lowest grade despite this imagery in my mind.

No sooner than two days after the "shock" I realized what my problem was. Or shall I say: what my problems WERE. I was able to determine three flaws in my character:

The first character flaw: playing the role of "everyone's savior"[9]. A person who plays this role thinks he/she has to help everyone under all circumstances. If the person chooses not to help somebody, then he/she will suffer from guilty feelings afterwards. Being afraid of these feelings of guilt, being an everyone's savior, tends to wear oneself out by helping and worrying about others.

The second character flaw: perfectionism or fear of failure. The other problem was closely connected with the lowest grade. This was MY FIRST failing grade. Something I was always so afraid of during my school and university years. I studied so carefully, the word "exaggeration" would be a mild way of putting it. The most ironic thing about this is that it was the fear of failure that sucked all the energy out of me, not the studying. It might not be a coincidence that I fell ill for the first time towards the end of my college years.

The third character flaw: playing the role of a people pleaser. I find it hard to say **No**. I am so afraid of other people's reactions that I just freeze and do nothing to defend myself. It is very difficult for me to stand up for myself. I find it hard to be angry at people that take advantage of me or hurt me. I tend to think of a reason why I should not stand up for myself, which of course is always an excuse. I became aware of this character flaw in seminars on emotional intelligence. However, if I look back at the story told above, I can see some traces of submissiveness in there too. It was not important that the student had disappointed me, for I had spent more time preparing language exercises for him than he had spent doing them. I only saw his misfortune, his failing grade. It was the end of the world for me, because the poor kid got the lowest grade. I also found that I had been trying too hard to make German lessons enjoyable for him. There was only **please him, him, him** and no **please me** in the story.

To sum up, I have found out that I have three character flaws that are most annoying and have nothing to do with my SchAD: trying to be **everyone's savior**, **perfectionism** or **fear of failure**, and last but not least, **being a people pleaser**. In other words, I want to please everyone and let everyone walk all over me if they choose to do so. I also impose myself on people in trying to help everyone. In addition to that, I want to be perfect at pursuing all these self-destructive strategies. Quite a deadly combination, right? Below you can read about how I went about eliminating some of the **everyone's savior**, **perfectionist**, and **people pleaser** in me. Join me in my journey to my new me: **the occasional helper**, **the predominantly diligent girl**, and **the dog that barks and sometimes also bites a bit**.

The Possibility of Character Flaw Improvements

We can go further. If the separation of your character from the symptoms of a mental illness is the first step, then the improvement of your character flaws can be the second step. When you improve your character flaws, there will only be the mental illness left to make your life miserable. Thus you will retain more energy for keeping your spirits up.

Let me warn you about some dangers on that matter, though. First, I wish to make it clear that I am not talking about **changing** one's character. I am only talking about **little improvements** that make one's life easier. For example, if someone tends to lose their temper too often and too intensively, they might think of reducing their outbursts a bit. On the other hand, I am a very submissive and silent person, for example, so I should learn to get a bit angry at least in situations where I am taken advantage of. In other words: I should learn how to stand up for myself.

In addition to that, I would also like to stress that we should learn to love ourselves the way we are first, and only then make improvements in our character. For an approach to improving ourselves that is too early and too aggressive could lead to self-hate. For two years, several times a day, I said to myself, out loud, 20 times in a row, **while looking into my eyes** in the mirror: "I love and appreciate myself". Only after two years of regular exercise did I start to explore my character flaws and blunt some of their sharpness.

Let me give you some examples from various personal growth seminars I have taken part in (you can find a complete list of all the seminars I have attended in the appendix). Here below the stories are organized according to my three character flaws, not according to the sequence of the seminars, however.

My first and third character flaws combined: playing both the role of everyone's savior and that of a people pleaser. In the spring of 2009 I attended a weekend seminar on improving one's self-image by basing it on self-reliance. The core of self-reliance – as the teachers showed us – is unconditional love and acceptance of oneself. However, as was shown to us, it is often the so-called **inner drives** that make us feel inadequate. Such drives are: **Be perfect! Please everyone! Hurry up! Be strong! Work hard! Everyone please me!**

As long as we follow these inner rules only in certain situations and to some reasonable extent, there is nothing wrong with them. If they totally overwhelm us, however, they become problematic. Or in other words: as long as we use them, it is fine. When they start using us, we feel trapped and subsequently develop a low self-image. We become perfectionists, people pleasers, etc.

These inner drives are ideals, and as such they are unreachable. If we identify ourselves with these ideals too much, the feeling of being "a loser" is very logical. Why? Because ideals are unreachable. We cannot really **Please everyone!** There are always people we cannot please. Also there are situations when the only sane thing to do is to help only ourselves. Imagine a woman, married to an alcoholic, that beats her. She finds it difficult to leave him, for he needs help. Yes he does, but she is in no position to help him. The only sane thing for her to do is to escape while she is still alive. Thus she should only help herself. I picked a tragic example to make my point, there are very ordinary situations that dictate the same course of action though. **Having the inner drive** *Please everyone!* is a very similar concept to **playing the role of a so-called people pleaser**. The difference between the two is that they come from different theoretical backgrounds.

Let me illustrate how **the people pleaser** in me turns on very easily. A little and seemingly unimportant thing "happened" to me at the above-mentioned seminar. We were working in pairs. Each partner was instructed to tell the other what one of his/her restraining beliefs was – in one sentence. Usually we have many such beliefs, but we had to pick one for the purpose of the exercise. The other person in the pair was supposed to ask their partner open questions, such as: "What exactly makes you think this way? Can you give me some examples from your past? Who told you should do this?"

I suggested that my partner start. She told me what her restraining belief was. I posed some questions and waited half a minute for her to really grasp the questions, as we had been instructed. Then she was supposed to listen to my restraining belief. Instead she started telling me a sad story that happened to her. In that moment my **Please-everyone** drive took over. I listened and encouraged her to tell me more by uttering a supportive sentence now and then. After a while the teacher said: "Time is up. Please finish the exercise slowly." Then I told my partner my belief in a hurry and she posed some open questions in a hurry too. I completely forgot about myself and listened to her, although we were not supposed to have a conversation.

You can guess what my restraining belief that I had chosen for this exercise was: "**I have to help everyone**." I was already aware of the fact that I tend to play the everyone's savior role at the time when this seminar took place, so I chose the sentence **I have to help everyone** as a restraining belief to work on in this pair exercise. The outcome of the exercise clearly showed that

I tend to play both the role of everyone's savior and the role of a people pleaser. I wanted to save my exercise partner by making supportive responses and I wanted to please her by listening to her, no matter what.

After the seminar I decided to do something about it. So now I have a new belief hanging on the wall next to the mirror in my bathroom: **I can choose whom to help.** It might seem stupid to those who can draw a healthy line in "the helping sphere". But it sure helps **me** to draw such a line.

And of course I try to practice drawing this line in real life too. The last two years I have been learning to stand up for my rights, to say "No!". I am still afraid of other people's reactions, but guess what – they seldom get upset, angry, or sad. Usually they just take it easy. There is another saying hanging on the wall of my bathroom: "It is my responsibility to set borders in a relationship. The other person's reaction is their responsibility. I **can** stand up for myself."

The incident at the above-mentioned seminar where I forgot about my needs and kept listening to the girl is a nice example of why we need mental work. Sayings hanging on our walls, sentences we keep repeating or rituals like cutting one's ties to a specific role according to the Phyllis Krystal method[10] are just examples of how we can start changing our thinking patterns. There are plenty of other approaches too.

When our brain needs re-programming, repeating sayings and visualizing symbols does the trick. It has for me. It was not enough to know that I play those dangerous roles. I needed to start re-programming my brain.

Obviously the obstacles in my mind were so strong that I had to find out from four different sources that I am not very good at getting angry. First it was the four temperaments we studied in the school for emotional intelligence: choleric, sanguine, melancholic, and phlegmatic. It turned out I most lacked the positive choleric characteristics of speaking up and standing up for myself, of fighting for my rights.

Later we studied the emotion of anger at the same school. We discussed two problematic types of dealing with other people or setting borders in relationships: **the swamp** and **the tractor**. Again, it turned out that I was the passive type anyone could walk over, i.e., **the swamp**, expecting others to "get it one day how they torture me, without me telling them". Soon afterwards, on a weekend seminar at the same school, I found out that I had a very strong **Please all!** drive, as I have already described above.

So obviously I had been suppressing anger for as long as I could remember, for it is my innate characteristic to be submissive. One of the last seminars I attended was that of Traditional Tibetan medicine[11]. I found out that also according to Tibetan medicine and philosophy I am prone to being submissive. I have too little **Tri-pa energy**, which is responsible for anger. Of course, here we are talking about low levels of righteous anger, not about explosive, rageful anger.

The Western world tends to think in terms of forces, atoms, subatomic parts, whereas the Eastern world has a long tradition of thinking in terms of the universal energy: qi, prana, etc. Yet if we read, for example, *The Field* by L. McTaggart[12], the East and the West seem to come together. It seems as if our traditional physical world and the Eastern world of energies are merging in our heads nowadays. Thus all this energy talk of the new age era should not scare you away. It is only a matter of time before official science is able to explain the energetic aspect of the human being. We can already film our aura (the bio-energy field surrounding our body) by Kyrlian photography however, thus there is no further need to prove that it exists.

My second character flaw: perfectionism or fear of failure.
The most helpful mental work on this matter is the mirror work described above, where I learned how to love myself just the way I am, all my mistakes included. I described this in detail in Chapter Two. I also recognized the role of the good little girl I was playing in a seminar held by P. Krystal and worked on that at that very seminar. I describe the Phyllis Krystal method in Chapter Four. I also do an exercise for reducing fear according to the method of P. Krystal whenever I am afraid of failure. In addition to that, I forgive myself for any failure, even if it is a stupid little thing. As stupid as it might seem, I find it helpful to say to myself out loud: "I forgive you, Helena." For as long as there is a feeling of guilt, there is also the need to forgive myself.

The Magical Power of Our Effort

The upper headline might sound a bit poetic, nevertheless, to sum the chapter up properly I only wish to stress that **Where there is a will there is a way**. And also that **If at first you do**

not succeed, try, try again. These are the two proverbs that keep me going in hard times when nothing else seems to work. Remember: If I managed to improve my well-being by starting to love myself, on one hand, and by making some adjustments to my character, on the other, so can you. **I let the psychiatrists deal with my mental illness and I dealt with my personality, to back up the efforts of the psychiatrists.**

It is true in many cases that **Where there is a will there is a way**. Nonetheless, our resistance to change as a person sometimes seems too strong to conquer. It resembles the force of gravity. The force of gravity is still a puzzle to physicists. The famous F_g remains very difficult to explain. And does not F_g resemble the secret force that seems to resist our efforts? We always have to put in a lot of effort if we want to improve ourselves or the world around us. As if the universe were somehow resistant to our will. We needed centuries to learn how to fly planes, for example. Were we fighting just the F_g or some other universal secret force that has no name?

Think of rich families. Very often the third generation becomes poor. There are many practical reasons why this happens. But maybe the common denominator would be that they are not capable of resisting the F_g like their parents and grandparents were, and everything "falls to the ground". They go out of business, get deep in debt, become alcohol or drug addicts, etc. Sometimes it is also the responsibility of their parents. They expect their children to become businessmen and businesswomen, so they put a lot of pressure on them and they break. Or sometimes the children have a totally different profession in mind, so they pursue a different career and the business of their parents slowly vanishes. There is nothing wrong with that, of course. I am just describing the process of becoming less well-off.

Speaking of effort, I have noticed that we often use the genetic aspect of our capabilities or our genetic predisposition for disease as an excuse for not taking action. For example: "I do not have the right genes for learning mathematics, so I will never finish school." or "My aunt smoked all of her life and died at the age of 92. She never had any serious health problems."

My answers would be: "So if your genes are not so brilliant, why don't you study harder?"

And: "So your aunt probably had no genetic predisposition for cancer or other illnesses caused by smoking. How can you be so sure you have the same DNA?"

Frankly I do not believe anything is purely genetic, except maybe the color of our eyes and our facial characteristics, and I also believe, on the other hand, that nothing is totally dependent on nurture. The **nature versus nurture** percentage of impact is an interesting research question for scientists, but does it really matter in our lives? It depends on how you look at it. I personally know that as long as there is a 1% genetic possibility for me to get well or to become a professional pianist, and if I desperately want to, I will give it a try.

I am **not** trying to say there is no point in developing the scientific research field of genetics. I am just encouraging you to act, learn, and persist, even if your genes do not give you "the best predisposition" to make things come true. Remember the famous quotation of Thomas A. Edison: "Genius is 1% inspiration and 99% perspiration."[13]

And do not forget about the universe. The universe is responding to your WISH – VISION – EFFORT triangle. For in addition to the force of resistance to change, there must also be another force helping us fulfill our mission in life. No matter what you call it, it works. Let me give you an example.

First I wrote the above sentence:

"I personally know that as long as there is a 1% genetic possibility for me to get well or to become a professional pianist, and if I desperately want to do that, I will give it a try."

A day after having written the above sentence there came an e-mail from a relative of mine with the subject: **E. Glennie**. She is one of the top classical percussion players, and is 95% deaf. What percent of her success can be attributed to her genes responsible for her "musical ear"? Being almost totally deaf, she chose to learn how to hear with her whole body instead.

Before this e-mail arrived I felt a bit uncertain about that bold statement of mine: "I personally know that as long as there is a 1% genetic possibility for me to get well or to become a professional pianist, and if I desperately want to do that, I will give it a try". However, after having received that e-mail I knew I was on the right track. For I deeply believe that there are no coincidences. The universe responded by backing me up.

To sum up – no matter how hard the task of improving the most annoying character flaws might seem, where there's a will, there's a way. I personally prefer to concentrate on the WISH – VISION – EFFORT triangle, rather than on the **nature versus nurture** dilemma. I am aware that my genes are my weaknesses and my potentials. That helps me not to exaggerate my efforts and get ill, on one hand, and not to neglect my talents, on the other hand. But I do not bother what the percentage of the genetic impact may be. I know that if there is a strong wish in me to improve myself, I first have to have a clear vision of how I want to improve. Then I have to put some effort into fulfilling my wish. When I put enough energy into this triangle, it seems to start rising in a spiral form, each corner stimulating the other two.

Reading books and realizing what useless thinking patterns we should get rid of is not enough to start changing. Just reading books on personal growth would be like finding out we are too fat, reading all possible books on dieting and physical exercise, but not actually changing our eating habits and not actually starting to exercise.

Our mind needs exercise just like our body does. And our mind needs some sweeping up, just like our body needs a shower. If we do not start cleaning out the mental garbage in our brains, we will become a burden to ourselves and the people we live or work with. Can you imagine coming to work smelling of 30-year-old sweat? That is similar to not doing any mental exercises whatsoever.

You will also look better if you feel happier. And the happiness comes from within. This is not just a phrase. No matter how many plastic surgeries you undergo, –you will never look like a specific famous actress, for example. Why not? Here are some reasons:

- An individual famous actress has a personality too. She is not just "the body of X. Y.". No plastic surgery can give you her personality. And personality transcends our skin. We may not all be able to see the aura of people, but we sure feel it. There is something about successful people we cannot really explain, isn't there? It could be their fine self-image for example. There is nothing wrong with plastic surgery if it only represents one thing you do about the way you look. However, if you put all your hopes and wishes on a poor plastic surgeon, you will be disappointed. For a plastic surgeon is no magician.
- Photography is art. Photographers of actresses and models look for their virtues not for their flaws. And of course there are many opportunities to cover up the little flaws later on the computer.

To sum up: What is wrong with adding about 20 minutes of meditation, affirmations, or visualizations to your daily routine anyway? You can take that time away from your sleeping hours if there is no other spare time. It will increase your quality of sleep. So you will not lose anything. Or you can watch 20 minutes less TV. But remember. This is a daily routine. Like taking a shower or brushing your teeth. It is not some weird new practice you will do for, let's say, three months, and then all of a sudden turn into some kind of guru or something like that. The question is: "Are you ready to start a different life? Are you ready to change only 20 minutes of your day radically in order to become happier?"

I sure hope your answer is **Yes**. For you have just said **Yes** to happiness.

CHAPTER FOUR

*Take the SchAD-bull by the horns
– Identify your present fears
and try to find their origin in your past
in order to finally eliminate them*

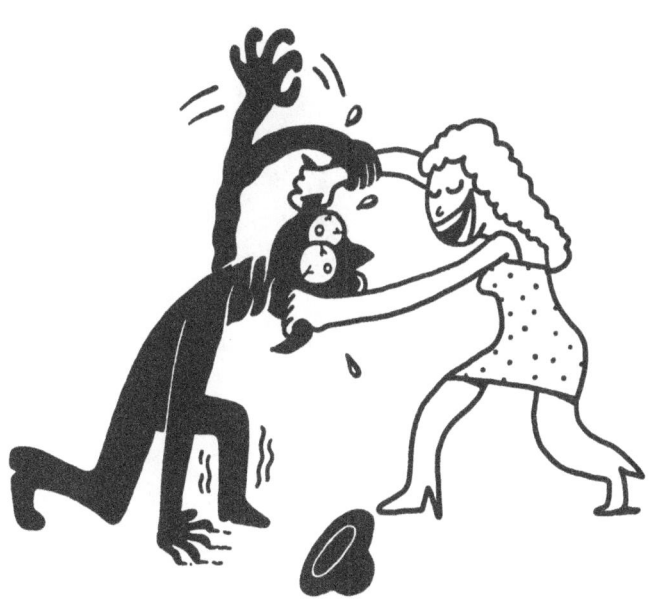

Warning

I wish to warn readers about two things here. **First, do not try to analyze your past without medical assistance.** The analysis itself could trigger an episode of SchAD, if you overdo it, and you can easily overdo it without the guidance of a psychiatrist. **Second, remember that not every fear has an origin in your past.** Some fears are merely biochemical irregularities in our brains. Again we need medical assistance to help us differentiate between the two types of fears: biochemical ones and "psychological" fears that originate from our past.

Psychologists may argue that "psychological" fears have nothing to do with one's mental illness, since the illness itself is biochemical. I would agree with this only partially. "Psychological" fears may well originate from some past events in your life. However, the mental illness itself makes those fears from our past worsen. Thus, if we manage to eliminate the "psychological" fears from our mind, the mental illness will lose some ground to stand on. That is also the reason why I chose the phrase **Take the bull by the horns** in the title of this chapter. The imagery of **a bull being taken by the horns** seems to fit very well into my dream of empowering mental patients to have control over their illness. There are various ways of identifying and eliminating the fears that have evolved in us because of our past experiences. I used the Phyllis Krystal method as described below.

The Real You
I came across an advertisement for a seminar held by Phyllis Krystal by chance. However, when I look back, the seminar came into my life at precisely the right time. Two years of regular daily mental work according to L. Hay's method had prepared me for the, in my opinion, slightly more analytical work advocated by P. Krystal.

Meditation presents a special issue for us – mental patients. I had heard in medical circles and also in alternative healing circles that some deep meditative methods can trigger a psychotic episode or some other serious mental health problems. Therefore I was cautious when trying new methods.

The imagery of the P. Krystal method could present a problem for people with SchAD, for it is very elaborated and it may evoke fear. Thus I would advise anyone who might be interested in the Phyllis Krystal method to:

1. First consult your psychiatrist and get a permission to join a P. Krystal method seminar.
2. Join at least one seminar before you start working by yourself at home. Do not try to work by yourself relying only on the books by P. Krystal. In her seminars Krystal always advises people with serious issues to work with a mentor. And you can meet a mentor at a seminar like this.

In exercises according to the P. Krystal method you will be able to connect with "the real you". Krystal uses a special term for this, but I do not wish to explain her method here, for that is not the purpose of this book. The most important thing to remember is that this "real you" is healthy. When you listen to "the real you", you do "the right thing" in life. You gradually find out that you need time for yourself, time for peace and quiet. In those moments you can meditate, walk alone in nature, or pursue a creative hobby. Through such activities you maintain the connection to the "real you". Connecting with your "real you" is a process to follow, not a goal to achieve. It is a way we go through life. The P. Krystal method definitely enhances this connection at great speed by cutting off the control of people and things over us.

Your "real you" is something very natural. It is not something to be so proud of in the sense that we think we are somebody special. Neither is it some weird thing "some meditating gurus are able to reach". Actually it is something very simple all children become aware of around the age of three, but they tend to gradually forget about it after starting to go to school[14].

Love, compassion, and acceptance of yourself and of others are also associated with your "real you". They reside in your heart. And they make your pain bearable. If you are connected with the "real you", it is much easier for you to accept the pain life thrusts upon you and to find your way through it. Also **the belief that in the long run everything that happens to us teaches us something** relieves some of the pain. This belief, in other words, is **the faith that the universe has the best intentions for us**.

An Example of Analyzing My Fears That Originate from My Past

The Story about My Miscarriage. In October 2008 I was lying in a bed at a gynecological clinic. I felt that a certain period of my life was over. I had a very strong feeling that the first "book" of my life was "opened to its last page". Then I simply began to write this book in reality. I took some paper and a pencil, sat in my bed at the clinic and used a magazine and my knees as the table to put the paper on. I was often interrupted by fellow patients and by nurses, but I felt an irresistible urge to write. These were my first paragraphs:

"October 11th, 2008. Saturday afternoon. Uterus cramps and heavy bleeding. Now it is certain. Our little embryo is dead. Sunday morning the doctors confirm the termination of the life that had begun 10 weeks ago. Monday morning they perform an operation on my uterus in order to clean it and thus prevent an inflammation.

My husband and I had just lost a baby actually. And I am calm. I – a psychiatric patient, diagnosed with schizoaffective disorder in 1996 – am calm. How come? Is it just the antipsychotic medication doing its work? No, it is also my thoughts. The pills calm the brain down, but they cannot change your personality from a pessimist to an optimist. For me this is a victory. I have changed.

But am I cured now? Can I live without pills? I think it is time to stop asking this silly question. I will take antipsychotic pills whenever my brain needs them. It is not just my psychiatrist, who represents Western medicine, who thinks I should control my disorder biochemically. Some months ago I read something very interesting in a book by His Holiness the **Dalai Lama**. He wrote that some types of anxiety and also some kinds of depression have a physical origin. Thus they can be successfully treated by medication[15]. This is in total accordance with what I found some weeks ago on the internet: "Schizoaffective disorder is a psychiatric diagnosis of neurobiological illness."[16] **Neurobiological** means connected to the nerves, the brain, and the biological processes inside those tissues. So it is my body that goes a little nuts at times, not my soul. All those years I thought I had a weak personality. Now I know there is no such thing as a weak personality. It is only a feeling you get, when your brain starts acting funny and you feel powerless, because you cannot control it."

A week after the surgery I got an inflammation of the uterus, so I was hospitalized again. I wrote my second set of paragraphs then:

"In the patient bed next to me there lies a 97-year-old woman. She reads newspapers without glasses, falls asleep for a while, then resumes reading. Then they take her to the operating room, perform an operation on her and bring her back. She falls asleep. After two hours they wake her up and she eats her whole lunch with care. Soon afterwards she gets up and walks out of the room. The doctor has sent her home, for she is fine. A physiological phenomenon? Maybe. Or is it her attitude combined with her exquisite physical health? She responded to all the information given to her by the nurses and doctor with an enthusiastic "Great!" and she kept expressing gratefulness for every little thing the nurses and doctor did for her. A broad mind and a grateful heart in an elderly body. A magnificent manifestation of the power of the mental aspect over the physical one.

On the common sense level I returned to the clinic because of an inflammation of my operated-on uterus. At first sight, this sounds like bad luck. But if I try to find some reason why this return to the clinic would be good for me, I cannot think of a better reason than the following: I came back to get to know this amazing elderly woman."

Two days later I found another bright side to the inflammation and wrote it down as well:

"I am still lying in the gynecological clinic. Luckily they are not going to perform another operation on my uterus. The operation they performed a week ago appears to have cleaned my uterus thoroughly after all.

I have also learned something here. I saw pregnant women take all sorts of medication. Now I know I can take a certain amount of antipsychotic medication the whole pregnancy, if necessary. Or should I say: my mind has finally grasped this fact. Thus there is a FEAR that is gone. The formula FEAR: F – false, E – evidence, A – appearing, R – real is coming true. My consciousness was not the problem – all my doctors, that is my personal doctor, the gynecologist, and the psychiatrist, had told me it would not be a problem if I had to take some antipsychotic pills during pregnancy. But my mind needed pictures."

The brightest side of the miscarriage, however, was a kind of inner peace in me. I finally got rid of a strange fear that had appeared every time I had spoken with the doctors. It did not happen over night, however. I had started exploring this fear a year prior to my stays at the gynecological clinic. Which leads us to another story, related below.

The Story about My Inner Child. In December 2007 I attended a weekend seminar on the Phyllis Krystal method in Switzerland[17]. In my meditations it was shown to me that my inner child had suffered a trauma in the maternity hospital where I had been born due to some undiscovered virus. This trauma happened soon after my birth. The mental work at the seminar helped us cure our inner child. In other words, the process of healing our psychological wounds was either started or accelerated – depending on the individual. The inner child is a psychological term. It usually stands for the playful aspect of our personality, on one hand, and for the painful memories from our childhood, on the other hand.

My mother told me years ago that in the first year of my life I had slept very poorly and vomited a lot. I was inspected by many doctors, but none of them was able to determine why this was happening. All these circumstances reported by my mother and the additional insight regarding the above mentioned meditation offered an explanation for my "primary fear" of doctors. By "nurturing" my inner child in daily meditations according to the P. Krystal method for a year starting from that seminar, I managed to eliminate the fear in me. The feeling of inner peace during my second stay at the gynecological clinic was proof of that.

Finding the Bright Side of Tragic Events

While analyzing the origins of my past fear of doctors I also learned a lot about the nature and dynamics of coincidence. This issue has always intrigued me and it still does. I have a very strong feeling that a pure coincidence is very rare.

Let me tell you two simple, everyday stories.

The story about the lady in a wheelchair. I went to the bus stop in front of our apartment building in order to catch a bus, but I was 20 minutes too early. It was raining and windy. Due to the low atmospheric pressure I felt very sleepy. So I said to myself: "Why don't I hop into the store round the corner and buy a package of coffee-filled chocolate pralines?" I went into the store and there I ran into the lady that I visit every week as a volunteer and chat with for an hour or two. She is in her 40s, but she lives in a local retirement home, for she cannot walk anymore. In the store I helped her pack the things she had bought into her backpack, hanging on the back of her wheelchair. This incident contributed some added value to the day – both mine and hers. I find it hard to see it as a pure coincidence.

The story about the shirt. I had been looking for a shirt as a birthday present for my husband for some weeks already when I finally managed to find an appropriate one, which I proceeded to buy. Then I stopped at a library on my way to the bus. I put the shopping bag on a shelf at the entrance of the library in order to be able to fold the umbrella. But then I forgot about the shirt in the shopping bag. After having read some newspapers, I left the library without it. I was already about 15 minutes away from the library when I realized that I had forgotten the shirt at the library. First I panicked, then I started visualizing the shirt at the entrance. And of course I hurried back. To my huge relief the shirt was still there. Was it a pure coincidence? By the way, it was a highly frequented library in the city center.

Let me go back to the beginning of this chapter. Was my spontaneous miscarriage a pure coincidence? I believe it was not. In my opinion, I first had to conclude the story about my dissatisfying job. I had to give my employer notice before I could become a mother. The "notice-still-to-be-given" was hanging over my head like the sword of Damocles. Let me explain.

When I got pregnant, the doctors gave me sick leave in order to reduce the stress. I played no tricks. I wrote a letter to the management saying I would probably take nine months of sick-leave for my risky pregnancy and that I had no intention of coming back after maternity leave either. I explained to my employer that I would give notice after my maternity leave, which lasts for a whole year in Slovenia.

In Slovenia when you are on sick leave for a longer period of time and also when you are on maternity leave, it is the state that pays your salary, not the employer. I felt I was somehow entitled to those 21 months of salary (9 months sick-leave for a risky pregnancy plus 12 months maternity leave), for I had been employed for 9 years. I figured in those 9 years I had contributed enough to the state budget, which would then be paying my salary for 21 months. I had been paying health insurance and maternity leave insurance during those years, for in our country this is mandatory if you are employed. The whole plan failed because of the spontaneous miscarriage. I could not find a reason to go back to work after the miscarriage. So I gave notice.

It might seem odd, but after the two stays in the gynecological clinic I felt relieved. I had had a weird feeling about the above-mentioned plan of staying on sick leave for nine months from the start. It would not have been a simple thing to do. I would have had to get confirmation from the health insurance institution every month. Which would have meant nine months of uncertainty for me.

I believe it all happened for the better. I am a supported wife now, which means that my husband pays my social and health insurance. I do not need any approvals for anything. I can get and be pregnant in the peace and quiet of my home. It is the only feasible way for me to have a baby. No matter what everyone had been telling me before. I have learned that I have to listen to myself.

Thus it seems that nothing is pure coincidence. Not even such a brutal thing as losing a child.

And maybe all these "bad" things **also** happened for another reason: so I could realize that I had finally gotten rid of my fear of doctors. Thus this spontaneous miscarriage somehow represents the end of the story that began when I was born.

My reconciliation with the past was rather simple, since the only "bad guy" was that virus that I had caught as a newborn baby. However, many times there are people involved – people that hurt us, people we have to forgive – if we want to move on.

CHAPTER FIVE

Taming your schizoaffective disorder – Practical tips for people with a mental illness

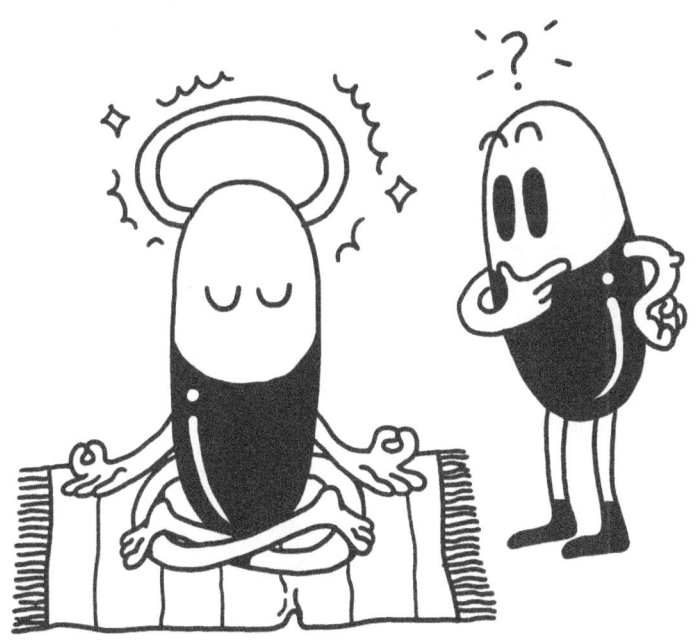

The Big Picture

Some time ago my husband and I were ascending a nearby hill. The path was steep. I got tired even before we had reached the peak. However, after the magnificent views opened up at the top of the hill, my fatigue vanished. I was delighted to be able to see "the big picture" of our town and neighborhood. It was a very clear day. One could see very far away. Only at that point did I understand how the landscape in the neighborhood was formed. I could see where our apartment building was situated and how you can get from one end of the town to the other.

The whole scene greatly resembled those moments in life when you see "the big picture" of your problem and thereby see the solution. It usually happens just before you would have given up. After months or even years of trying to figure a way out of a difficult situation, suddenly there is new hope. Sometimes you find new information that helps you solve the problem in a book or on the internet. Sometimes a specific new person comes into your life who is able to help you or show you the way. Or something else happens that helps solve the problem.

For example, I had wanted to live without antipsychotic medication for years. I thought: "If I can live without medication, it means I am cured." I did not want to accept my mental illness. Thus I did not accept the medication either. However, about two years ago I finally accepted my schizoaffective disorder. I felt so relieved that I wanted to write a book about my experiences with this mental illness. So I started writing the book in October 2008. While writing this book I always felt as if I was on the top of a hill. I saw "the big picture", which enables me to write by reading many self-help books, by attending self-help seminars. And also by analyzing my personality, my past, and by doing a lot of mental exercises, all of which I learned in the books and seminars listed at the back of this book.

Many people write about the importance of being as well informed about our illness as possible. I could not agree more. All I can add is something I have read in a famous book by H. C. Cutler and His Holiness The Dalai Lama XIV[18]. **The Dalai Lama states that there are three causes of suffering. Ignorance is one of them.** So enjoy researching in order to see "the big picture" of your situation. This will make it easier for you to find a solution to the problem.

Why me?

I would like to say something about the classic question that comes along with one's first mental illness episode: **Why me?** I can laugh about it today, but this was a very serious question 14 years ago, when I had my first psychotic episode. It seemed sooooooo unfair. My brain was constantly producing self-pitying questions: "What have I done to deserve this? Is this a punishment? For what? Have I not been taking good care of my health? Why has this happened precisely to me and not to somebody else? My classmates are finishing their studies, some are already married. Some have already been promised a job. And here I am – my studies not finished, single, no job prospects, no boyfriend prospects. I'm doomed."

Well, everyone has had bad moments of self-pity. That is

normal. The problem with my self-pity was that this "mode" was "on" 24 hours a day, 365 days per year, for 7 years. In the meantime I had finished my Bachelor of Arts degree. I had gotten a job and had met my future husband, nevertheless the "self-pity-mode" was still "on".

How is this possible? It is called **thinking patterns.** One gets into the habit of self-pity and that is how it stays, even if the outer-world situation changes. Eventually, in the summer of 2004, I decided to change my "inner-world situation", as I have mentioned several times already. I was encouraged by my boyfriend's friend, who lent me the above-mentioned book by L. Hay[19]. I started reading. It did not seem to work. I started doing the mental work described in the book. It did not seem to work either.

I said to myself: "I have hit rock bottom. I am constantly thinking of committing suicide. I cannot fall any deeper. I will continue the affirmations and visualizations. They have to start working one of these day." I was stubborn as hell and so I persisted. Twice a day for about 20 minutes. The first results began to show after a year. They were not real results that one could describe. I just began to feel a bit better.

And so I went on with the mental work. In the summer of 2005 I added another exercise recorded on a set of audio cassettes by L. Hay[20]. Actually there are two 20-minute long meditations on the last cassette in the set. I was listening to the same two meditations for two years. Each evening one or the other helped me fall asleep.

In 2006 I started working according to the method of Phyllis Krystal on a daily basis. I have not stopped visualizing according to this method up until today. I have also continued to do the mirror work according to the L. Hay method up until today. In addition to that, I joined a school for emotional intelligence in 2008, where we underwent a great deal of self-analysis, psychological tests, group and pair drama games, and of course visualizations and affirmations. You will find a more precise overview of my daily routine from 2004 until today towards the end of the book.

Today, after six years of working on my ways of thinking, I can say that I have changed.

It is either the hard way or no way. It is your choice. But do not worry – after a few years of mental work, you begin to like it so much that you cannot stop doing it.

We should view our sensitive brain as a precious jewel.

I view my brain as a precious jewel that helps me not repeat my past mistakes. I see my brain as an alarm light. When I am too stressed out, the light switches on. It is important for me not to panic. I stop, analyze the last few days, determine what the stress factors have been. Then I try to avoid them. However, sometimes there are factors you cannot avoid. In that case, the only thing that can help is to see your doctor, who will usually prescribe a higher dosage or maybe add some other medication to your regular medication. I believe I will live longer precisely because of SchAD, for it helps me avoid stress.

Is schizoaffective disorder an illness of the soul or one of the body? My view of the dilemma.

I can say from my personal experience that this disease is very biochemical. I had been writing a diary for a few years and together with my psychiatrist we determined that my symptoms worsen before I get my period. So hormones are affecting the biochemicals in my brain. I also remember that every time I was hospitalized I got my period in a locked ward, which is the first type ward they put you in. Thus premenstrual syndrome always added to it.

This is my personal view. I came to this opinion gradually. At first – when I was still in denial – I hated pills and I thought that my mental illness was only a matter of my injured soul and should be treated accordingly. Later I became grateful that the medication always worked for me and stabilized me relatively quickly. I still believe my soul was injured. But I would never have made it so far without the biochemical imbalances in my brain having been cured by means of antipsychotic medication. I believe it was the combination of taking care of my body and my soul that made it possible for me to get well. So, in my opinion, if Western medicine concentrates more on the body (the natural biochemistry of the brain plus medication), there is nothing wrong with alternative medicine approaches concentrating more on the soul. I personally believe that so-called integrative medicine (Western medicine plus alternative medicine) should be our goal in the future.

Nonetheless, I would advise you to be careful with such philosophical questions as **Is a mental illness an illness of the soul or of the body?** For in my opinion, philosophy is like medicine: If you take too much of it, it is poisonous.

Fighting on Many Fronts: Western Medicine, Mental Exercises, Natural Healing, Lifestyle Choice

Surely you have been faced with the classic and also very annoying dilemma: Should I use Western medicine, for example pills, or should I try alternative medicine approaches?

I say this is no dilemma at all. My suggestion would be: Do both at the same time. And tell your psychiatrist about all your activities. Form a team with your doctor, do not be afraid of him/her. The psychiatrist is on your side.

The fear of psychiatrists may seem funny to people that have never experienced anxiety or paranoia themselves. However, such fearful thoughts are actually very common among people with schizoaffective disorder. I had them myself. Such thoughts are totally baseless, of course. So try to just let them go. Do not take them seriously. They are just some biochemical irregularities in your brain.

Biochemical level of treatment. Western medicine medication heals our brain on the biochemical level rather successfully. However, there are some problems too. Apart from the side effects, there is also the fear of antipsychotic pills or injections. I was afraid of the pills I was taking too. Thoughts like the following kept popping up in my mind:

- "I will get addicted."
- "I will get fat."
- "The pills make me feel like a vegetable. I am not in contact with my feelings."

Now, there might be some truth to these three sentences. Who knows what science might be able to prove 20 years from now. However, we need to deal with schizoaffective disorder right now. So let us be practical. I suggest you keep taking the pills and ignore such thoughts – like I do. Try to just let go of thoughts of this kind. Do not take them seriously. Do not fight them. They will resist. Just let them go. Imagine they are clouds and watch them go away.

Even if such thoughts are true to some extent, there is nothing we can do about them. We need the pills to make us function normally in life: get up, eat, work, have fun, talk sensible things to the people around us, sleep. In my opinion, however, in order to be truly happy some day in the future , you need other supportive methods to back up the medication. I would like to advise you again: Always consult your doctor first regarding all other methods you are interested in trying before actually trying them! And do not continue using a method that makes you feel strange or gives you sleeping disorders. It might not be the right one for you. Explore, but be cautious.

There is no alternative medicine method appropriate for all human beings with the same health problem. Just as there is no such Western medicine pill. As you know, there are many slightly different pills for schizoaffective disorder. Your doctors sometimes have to try different types of antipsychotic medications before they can say which one is best for you. The one that was best for me, for example, caused my friend with schizoaffective disorder to put on 88 pounds in a few months. Now she naturally takes some other type of antipsychotic pills.

Usually doctors are lucky if they can get it right the first time. It is because each human being is so unique. There are some rules, but there are also many exceptions. The exceptions make life difficult but also interesting.

Another common fear among people that get a mental illness is the idea that because the doctors are trying various pills, they might be using the patient as a subject in an experiment. Another totally false idea of course. Sometimes even the relatives of patients adopt this idea. Again – ignore the idea. Do not take it seriously. The people who actually participate in experiments do so as volunteers. Your psychiatrist is not doing anything behind your back.

You must also know that doctors are not allowed to prescribe alternative treatments unless such treatments have been proven scientifically. This will make it easier for you to understand why they might not exactly encourage you to try alternative medicine methods. Have patience. Take one step at a time.

Mental exercises or mental work. When a mental illness episode is over and you are stabilized, you and your psychiatrist might try some cognitive-behavioral therapy and see if it does not disturb your brain too much. It worked for me.

My psychiatrist was a bit reluctant at first, but it did no harm to me and eventually it helped a lot. I started to view my SchAD as a biochemical problem of my brain thanks to **cognitive-behavioral therapy (CBT)**. An analysis of the notes in my CBT diary also showed that my depression and anxiety worsen before my menstrual period.

It was very important for me to come to the conclusion that it is really the natural biochemicals in my brain that "think all the nonsense". It is the little molecules that are "stupid", not **me**. So I started to view the silly thoughts like little molecules in my brain. I could not just send them away. The thoughts resisted. The more I tried **not** to think about committing suicide, for example, the more the suicidal thoughts were present. So I started to take them less seriously. I just watched them. I let them "think themselves out." I kept telling myself: "The thoughts that have to be thought will be thought. I will wait for them to calm down. I took the pills. They must work eventually. I'll wait." Just like you patiently wait for a little child to calm down, when you know there is nothing else you can do for the child.

Thus eventually the depressive and the anxious thoughts ceased. It took me three years, though. I was doing my CBT homework regularly and I always discussed it with my psychiatrist when I went to see her once a month.

The relationship between psychiatrist and patient is a very complex thing. I will probably never understand it fully. However, as a patient I have come to a conclusion that is very important in my opinion. I believe it helps if we view ourselves to be as clever as our psychiatrists. It might seem too bold of me to say a thing like that, but let me explain. The psychiatrist has enormous theoretical knowledge and also broad knowledge of differences between individual patients. On the other hand, I as a patient am the only one that is "with myself" 24 hours a day. In other words: I can observe myself all the time, whereas my doctor cannot. Thus, in my opinion, the winning combination is to combine the general knowledge of the psychiatrist and my knowledge of what is going on in my mind 24 hours a day. This manner of thinking also eliminates the very common feeling of being subordinate to the psychiatrist, which usually evokes anger in the patient and is thus not constructive.

In order to be able to provide the psychiatrist relevant information we should get in the habit of observing ourselves. This is not easy. But we can try. A useful suggestion might be to keep a diary with short notes like: "slept well" or "slept for only two hours", "felt sad" or "felt too happy", which is the basis for CBT. If we show such a diary to our doctors, they will be able to discern some patterns. As mentioned above, my psychiatrist was able to determine that my symptoms worsen just before my period. Subsequently this observation has helped me, because I do not take myself very seriously the week before my period. I know it is the hormones that are disturbing my brain and making me behave badly. It is not me as a personality that is annoying and difficult. I also tell my husband not to take me seriously the week before my period. It helps our relationship a lot.

By making short notes of our activities we can also find out what the triggers of our symptoms are. For example: "stayed out late" and "had trouble falling asleep" one after the other in the diary could suggest we had better go to bed early.

In addition to the above mentioned CBT I also applied various alternative approaches which are described in other chapters of this book: affirmations according to L. Hay, P. Krystal's method, the school for emotional intelligence. These approaches are considered alternative medicine, whereas CBT is an official Western medicine approach.

Natural Healing. This is considered alternative medicine. There is a bio-energy field surrounding our body that is called aura and which can be filmed by a special camera – a Kyrlian camera. There are some scientists exploring it, but usually they are not taken seriously by the majority of scientists. Natural healers work predominantly on the bio-energy level.

In 2009 I was treated by a Great Reiki Master Teacher (5th, 6th, and 7th levels of reiki). He does holistic healing, reiki, hatmara (biotransformations, biorgonomy), magnified healing, sound baths with gongs, pranotherapy, and radiostesy – all considered alternative medicine approaches or natural healing. I visited him twice. First he treated me and then he said I must have a mild variant of schizoaffective disorder. He also pointed out that schizophrenia in general is curable. This reiki master said that "it is the self-programming of patients with schizophrenia that does the most damage". In other words: we keep telling ourselves we are ill. Another word for it is also autosuggestion.

He told me that I had managed to remove all the negative thinking patterns typical of schizoaffective disorder by doing mental work. The bio-energy aspect of the disease was still causing me insomnia though. This **bio-energy healer** helped me with my bio-energy flow. He also told me to drink fish oil and eat more meat, especially fish and white meat to help my brain recover. In addition, he recommended using predominantly olive oil in the kitchen. Thus later I got used to eating more meat. And I underwent fish oil therapy for half a year.

Change of Lifestyle. In 2009 I also registered for a seminar on Traditional Tibetan Medicine to broaden my knowledge. I thought I was only going to get to know some basics of Tibetan medicine. It was during the first day of lectures that I learned that the lecturer was offering individual appointments. I applied for one. After inspecting me, he gave me a massage and taught my husband how to do it regularly at home. The massage with hot oil seems to help. When my husband presses on certain points of my body with a Tibetan herbs bag soaked in hot oil, I feel excessive energy leaving my body. After the massage I feel extremely relaxed.

In addition to the massage, the Tibetan medicine doctor also advised me to **change my lifestyle**. He told me to eat more meat, less fresh salad, more soup, especially chicken soup. He advised me to listen to soft music with low tones, do light meditation and yoga, take short hikes (lower mountains), etc. It is interesting that I intuitively did all that, except for the diet instructions. Only I felt lazy for not hiking in higher mountains and not jogging anymore like I used to. Now I feel fine. The feeling of guilt is gone.

The Tibetan doctor also told me: "When you lie in bed, tell yourself: 'It is time for bed. Stop thinking.'" He added: "I used to think about my patients at night, but I learned to discipline my mind later." I asked him: "So are you trying to tell me that I can learn to obey my order to myself: 'Time for bed!'? It is a habit, right?" He said: "Yes." That felt great. And now I am really able to put my mind to sleep by repeating silently: "Time for bed. No more thinking. Just exist." It might sound childish, but I really thought I was not able to tell my mind to stop thinking until just recently. Again we are talking about self-programming here.

Let me tell you how I have changed my lifestyle in order to sleep better. Sleeping disorders or more precisely insomnia were always the first symptom of my schizoaffective episodes. Thus over time I became afraid of not being able to fall asleep in the evening, which could be the first sign of a SchAD episode. This fear made it even more difficult for me to fall asleep. Therefore I started observing myself and in a few years I have come to the following conclusions, which were also supported by the Tibetan doctor's suggestions:

1. I should go to bed at 11 p.m. the latest.
2. I should not work or have an exciting conversation after 7 p.m. Evening parties are to be avoided.
3. I should not work on weekends.
4. If the day is stressful, I need relaxation activities in the evening: Tibetan massage, incense, Tibetan herb tea or chamomile tea, soft instrumental music.
5. After the relaxation techniques, I should just lie down and keep repeating silently in my head:

"Just exist." or "It is time to sleep."
6. When my thoughts get very annoying, I imagine
   they are clouds drifting away from me.
   I do not try to fight against them.

I am usually successful and fall asleep before midnight. Of course this is the result of a combined treatment: **Western medicine (antipsychotic medication), mental exercises (CBT, the L. Hay and P. Krystal methods), natural healing (occasional reiki, regular Tibetan massage), a change of lifestyle (according to the advice of the Tibetan medicine doctor).**

You have changed your way of thinking into a more positive one, but now you feel uncomfortable about it – what to do?

I would like to warn you about the principle of resistance. I remember that after four years of mental work I had managed to remove the worst "garbage" from my mind. And I should have felt happy. Yet I did not. It actually felt odd not to be worried all the time any more. My consciousness worked like a mine-sweeper. I was constantly looking for something I could worry about. I knew there was nothing to worry about, but I still somehow wanted to keep worrying. It is called the power of habit. I was so used to being worried all the time that it felt odd to be carefree. Luckily I have read in various books about this resistance in our minds. Thus I persisted with my new ways of thinking. Slowly the "mine-sweeper-program" was shut down. What a relief!

Choose the people you hang out with.
I learned that I must carefully choose the people I hang out with. All normal people do. However, once you have been diagnosed with a mental illness you can easily lose all friends. Then you might think that anyone who wants to hang out with you does so out of pity, so you gladly accept anybody's company. However, people that are very different from you can take the last remaining energy out of you. Let me tell you my story about friends.

When I fell ill for the first time, my friends tried to stick with me at first. Nonetheless, after a while it got too hard for them to look at somebody who was quiet all the time and looked like a walking corpse. I did not say it out loud, but they must have felt I was thinking of suicide a lot. Today I am glad they limited their contact with me to a few times a year. They had to do it for their own protection, for a bad mood is contagious, as you well know. It would have worn them out.

When I met my future husband, I had practically no friends, so I attached myself too much to him. It was not the best thing to do, but the way I see it from today's perspective, it was the only way for me at that time. He stood by me no matter what. He helped me become who I am today. I would not have made it without him.

It was much later that I came out of my fear and depression jungle to such an extent that I was able to renew my old friendships and even make new ones. However, I came across another danger – the belief that I had to accept anyone as a friend. I thought I was not supposed to be choosy about new friends, since I had been "alone" for such a long time. My husband and I also moved to another town, so I had little contact with my old friends. Soon I realized that my new friends who were very different from me were only exhausting me. I realized I had to become choosy, or I would fall ill. Today I have two new friends in the town we moved to. I mean that kind of friend you see every week. Thus I am not that terribly tied to my husband anymore.

Another trap I fell into was "analyzing my relatives". After having acquired a lot of knowledge about personal growth in various seminars, books, and daily mental work, I suddenly wanted to help everyone. This was exhausting too. So I had to reduce family visits.

It was this winter that I finally managed to find the balance between solitude and socializing. When I feel there has been too much talk with my friends, I simply take some days off and enjoy the peace and quiet of our home or take a stroll in the forest. As far as my relatives are concerned, I try to accept them the way they are. I just listen and make as few remarks as possible. When listening to them still stresses me out, my dear husband gives me a Tibetan heat compress massage before going to bed. This makes keeping the balance between solitude and socializing much easier.

I do love people and wish everyone the best, but I am very sensitive to the energy they send out, that is why I am a bit of a loner. Of course it is predominantly the negative energy that people send out that gives me sleeping disorders. But also a huge amount of positive energy in the evening makes it harder for me to fall asleep. That is why my home sweet home became a sort of "headquarters of peace". A quiet place only for me and my beloved husband, no loud music, no TV. It is a place where we both refuel our "tanks" with life energy. Once a week we also get a major refill in the mountains or by walking around a lake.

And last but not least I wish to address the problem of negativity. I have an acquaintance who likes complaining. It's her habit, her attitude, and her way of life. To my great surprise she noticed pretty soon that I don't really like this attitude of hers. And guess what – she started telling jokes and developed a new habit. Now she jokes in my presence almost all the time. And I surely like that a lot.

The point I am trying to make here is the following: People that keep complaining and therefore take a lot of energy from you are not doing it on purpose. They are not even aware of what they are doing. Thus be gentle and diplomatic in showing them the way to a more positive approach to life. Making jokes can be useful, because laughing can catch on and last while you are with the person.

In addition to that, I would like to warn you that some people will fight very hard to keep their negativity, for in their world negativity is all they have. In such cases you have to take care of yourself first and protect yourself by avoiding them to some extent.

Of course I only became "allergic" to pessimistic and complaining people after having successfully changed myself. On the other hand, when I was still a lamenting pessimist myself, I never noticed anything wrong with being negative.

Humor also cheers up those who suffer from a mental illness. It makes it easier for us to accept our illness. While surfing the internet I recently found a number of very cool standup comedians who try to make mental illness more casual by making jokes about it:
http://www.standupformentalhealth.com/.

The Importance of Listening to People Who Live with Us and Care about Us

I write about the importance of self-observation above. Nonetheless, sometimes we are in denial. We get the usual symptoms, but we think we are all right. This is the time when people who live with us can help. It is very helpful if we live with at least one person we can trust as this person can tell us that we are behaving in an unusual way. The changes in mental health can be very rapid, that is why I am talking about people who live with us and thus see us every day, and not about relatives or friends in general.

I have often read on various internet sites that the people we live with do not understand us. Sometimes this can be true. Sometimes, however, we can get this feeling because we are in denial. Thus our goal could be to learn to differentiate between two separate cases: 1. The people we live with really do not understand us. 2. The people we live with are trying to warn us about the worsening of our mental health, but we are not ready to listen.

By listening to our partners, parents, siblings, etc., we can show them that we trust them. This will make them feel good and they will take even better care of us. I know there are people who do not have anyone they can trust. All I can say is I hope that they meet somebody nice. For mental illness can really be a pest if you face it all alone.

In October of 2003 my last schizoaffective episode set in. It was my third one. But for my husband it was the first one he observed. It was a shock for him to see somebody completely lose their mind. Especially because that somebody was me – his girlfriend at that time. I could have prevented this episode by admitting to myself that I was manic. Instead I chose to be "too clever" and not to listen to anyone – neither to my psychiatrist, nor to my future husband. It only dawned on me that I needed antipsychotic pills when I started imagining I was the second Jesus Christ. Then I was put in a locked ward of a psychiatric clinic willingly and I took all the medication without resistance. I stayed in the locked ward for only a few days. Then the doctors let me spend the weekend with my husband, for he assured them that I was behaving a lot better after having received the proper medication at the clinic. I spent another two months in an unlocked ward, but kept going home on weekends.

This story could have been the last chapter of our relationship. Instead we survived as a couple. I also learned to listen to him when he warns me of my early symptoms. I always see my psychiatrist soon enough to prevent an episode. My willingness to listen to my husband is one of the reasons I can call the 2003 episode the last I have experienced.

When should you tell people about your mental illness?

I know mental illness can be a burden. While surfing on the internet I came across the following question many times: "Should I tell people at work about my illness?"

My answer would be: First, pick a job you know you **can** handle. Second, do not tell anyone at first. Let them get to know you as you are first. They might look at you through "the wrong glasses" if your mental condition were the first thing they know about you. Later you will see how things evolve. You can certainly tell the colleagues at work you start trusting.

The only problem might be if your potential boss asks you already during the first job interview very directly: "Are you healthy?" Now, this question is not necessarily offensive. Some businesses are so small they cannot afford too many people going on sick leave. I personally would tell the truth, but that is only because I do not know how to lie. I would get caught, so I do not lie – I am too lazy for that.

I know there are laws in certain countries that forbid the employers from asking job candidates about their health. However, the law is one thing, respecting it is another. Thus you had better be prepared for the nasty question: "Are you healthy?" Sometimes the employer is trying to protect you too. Why on earth would you want to be hired for a job that is going to deteriorate your health, make you quit, and leave you with the sense of being a loser? Speaking for myself, I would never apply for a job that includes working at night, for instance. This is my limitation and I intend to respect it. In order for the biochemistry in my brain to remain stable, going to bed at 10 or 11 p.m. is crucial. If I experiment with my sleeping hours, I get insomnia, which can easily lead to a schizoaffective disorder episode.

If you decide not to answer this nasty question truthfully and your employer finds out later that you have an illness, please tell them the truth then. You can put it this way: "I was afraid to tell you the first minute we met. It is not easy to talk about a serious illness." And remember: Not all employers have a heart of stone. And even more important: A mental illness or a physical illness are equally uncomfortable. Illness is illness.

What about your first date with a "love-relationship candidate"? I would say – fire away. The sooner you get rid of those who have too strong prejudice regarding mental illness, the better. I had scared off quite a few guys before meeting my husband. I am glad I had. Working for somebody is one thing. One can manage to be fully in control of one's emotions at work, but your illness will show sooner or later at home. Your life partner will have to be willing to try to cope with it. It helps if you are a team from the start.

There are some exceptions in life and a job interview is such an exception. However, in general in most cases in life I believe the truth significantly resembles a waxing depilation. It hurts like hell, but the pain does not last very long and you feel great when you leave the beauty salon or your bathroom.

Little Innocent Addictions of Every Day Life

Watching TV is like eating sugar. Once you start, you cannot stop. It is an addiction. We all know that. My husband and I do not have a TV set, for we never felt the need to buy one. We find all the necessary information on the internet. We choose what we want to watch, hear, or read and we are not exposed to all the commercials telling us what we really want.

Similarly, we have reduced our sugar intake to a minimum – a few pieces of dark chocolate per day, for sugar can be an addiction too. I bake apple strudel using only cinnamon – I do not add any sugar. My mother-in-law makes stewed fruit for us using no sugar either. We like to add fresh fruit to the stewed ones and prepare delicious fruit salads.

When my husband and I happen to sit down and watch TV at my parents' house for hours now and then, or when we eat a lot of sweets at Christmas, for example, we have a strange feeling. The feeling that we have spoiled something. Because we have gotten used to living almost without sugar or TV. It is all a matter of habit. We choose our habits. They are not written in our genes.

In addition to that, it is not just the amount of time you spend watching TV. It is also the content you watch. You surely do not want to watch shows that reinforce the old thinking patterns you want to get rid of. So be active in front of your TV set and carefully choose the shows you watch.

Saying Thanks as a Habit

In addition to giving up bad habits, it is also useful to adopt new ones. I am learning to be grateful, for instance. I say 'thanks' very often. Let me give you some examples. The following paragraphs were written in autumn 2008 when I gave notice at work:

"The first day of freedom – I gave notice. I have quit a so-called 'safe job'. A job you can hardly lose, but one you also only get rid of with difficulty. Why with difficulty? Because you have to have guts to do so. Everyone around you is telling you to reconsider. Or at least to find another job before you quit. For me it was enough to have my husband supporting me on this decision. I took my chances. I am not looking for another job now. I need peace and quiet. I need time to study what I am really interested in: new age psychology and philosophy. This is the field in which I really want to make a living some day.

I need a break from the classic life: a job plus some spare time. And of course I want to get pregnant and give birth under as little stress as possible. I will minimize the possibility of a psychotic episode during pregnancy by being unemployed and thus avoiding the stress of work. I told everyone I was going to open a private company and give German lessons. Instead I am studying again and writing a book. Only my husband knows my secret.

Today I really feel free. I never felt so at ease in my whole life. So relaxed and freed from the past. A moment worth living for. And what was the lesson from those nine years of an unsatisfying job? I had to learn how to say 'no'. I tried to give notice five years ago, but it was not accepted. I had to do it the right way this time.

Thank you god, or the universe, ... for the support of my husband in giving notice, for his emotional support and for his financial support ... thank you for putting these words into my husband's mouth: "Do not worry about your income when you give notice. Just keep doing what you really enjoy doing. I will take care about the money we need to live a normal life."

Thank you god... for letting me discover my true mission in life. Up until this autumn of 2008 I had not known **what on earth I wanted to do in my life as an occupation**. Now I do know. I want to help people by writing books.

Thank you god... for letting me discover a more important income than money, the income called love.

And last but not least … thank you god for letting me cut the ties to my former job …

for cutting them physically on the 17th of March, for that was the last time I set foot in my former office, and it was my husband who tidied up my office the day before yesterday…

for cutting them rationally in March …

for cutting them financially last week …

for cutting them emotionally yesterday, when I made a list of the professional books from my former office I wanted to give away.

I wanted to give all my personal books to my employer, but they would not accept them. My husband tried to explain to them that I am not going to need them anymore, but it was in vain. Now I have a six-foot row of books in our little apartment. First I was angry at my employer, for they could well use the books for their purposes. But then I tried to make peace with what had happened. Yesterday I made a list of the books with all the bibliographic data, including the ISBN and ISSN numbers and now I will try to find some institution that might want them. I am looking forward to being able to give."

A few days later, still in autumn of 2008, I wrote the following paragraphs:

– "It is Christmas Eve and since there is no coincidence – I gave the books from my former office to a library today. I feel so grateful for having found somebody that needs the books. It is such a 'Christmas spirit feeling'. "

– "The strangest thing happened to me the other day. I was eating rice with vegetables in a hurry. All of a sudden I started to feel that the food in my esophagus had stopped going down. First I tried to reach for a glass of water, but then I stopped breathing, so I panicked and ran to the neighbors' apartment. I thought: "If I faint because of a lack of oxygen, the neighbors can call an ambulance." Just before reaching their bell, I vomited and started breathing again.

Just a silly incident? No, it was a lesson. I used to have a feeling I was slow at working. So I constantly hurried – even when eating. It gradually became a habit of literally throwing food into my stomach. It looks like I will have to break the habit now. Since that rice meal I take a few deep breaths before I start eating, I say thanks for the food and wish myself bon appétit even if I eat alone."

Keep your spirits up!
My advice to those of you who are diagnosed with a mental illness would be: "Whatever you do, never give up totally."

I would like to say something about so-called suicidal thoughts. I believe they are caused by biochemical imbalances in the brain. But I also believe that they can become a habit. So developing more optimistic thinking patterns can help even in "bad biochemical times".

And to all the healthy people who are reading this book, I would like to say the following. If you happen to know anyone who is currently staying in a psychiatric hospital, do not hesitate to visit them. You might end up saving a life.

EPILOGUE

**Failure is not an option.
Says who?**

Have you ever felt that you have failed (badly) in your life?

I could say I have failed. I have failed to make a career as a scientific researcher. After years of studying to become a researcher, all of a sudden an illness struck me. It was schizoaffective disorder and I could not believe it. I somehow came through the first three episodes. However, the illness and working day after day in an uncomfortable environment made me say goodbye to my career dreams at the age of 34.

Some people think one has to reach the peak of their career between 30 and 40 years of age, for after 40 one starts to get old. Now I am beginning a whole new profession – helping others based on the experiences I went through. I do not plan to start getting particularly old at the age of 40. Actually, I plan to be a peak performer as a self-help writer and a motivational speaker sometime around 50. Now at 36 I probably still have 60 more years to live, which means that I have time.

I also do not care if I fail, because in all these years of struggling with my schizoaffective disorder, I have learned to fail properly. To rephrase **Frank Sinatra**'s song **My Way**, I bit off more than I could chew, but then again, I ate it up all by myself. Or if I put it in modern new age terms: I made my decisions, I took action, and I accepted all responsibility for my actions. And frankly speaking: I do not care if I fail, since I can always say I did my best.

I have learned that blaming somebody else for your failures is not an option. One has to take responsibility for one's life. However, failure **is** an option, because sometimes you have to admit defeat.

MY DAILY ROUTINE

The following table of my daily routine in the last 6 years is not a precise chronicle. It is an outline that should give the reader a general impression of what I have done and do in "my moments of the day". Where there is no frequency (once a week, etc.) it means I did it or do it almost every day.

	morning	throughout the day	evening
2004 (2nd half)	The Five Tibetan Rejuvenating Exercises (FTRE), Hay visualizations	(at work) Hay mirror work, when I went to the restroom	Cognitive Behavioral Therapy (CBT), Hay visualizations
2005	FTRE, Hay visualizations	(at work) Hay mirror work, when I went to the restroom	CBT, Hay audio cassette guided meditation (second half of 2005)
2006	FTRE, PhyllisKrystal visualizations (PKV)	(at work) Hay mirror work, when I went to the restroom	CBT, Hay audio cassette guided meditation
2007	FTRE, PKV	(at work) Hay mirror work, when I went to the restroom	CBT (first half of 2007), volunteer work once a week (second half of 2007), painting and drawing course once a week, Hay audio cassette guided meditation (first half of 2007), PKV – the tree visualization (second half of 2007)
2008	FTRE, PKV	(at work) Hay mirror work, when I went to the restroom	volunteer work once a week, oriental dance once a week, PKV – the tree visualization
2009	FTRE, PKV	(working at home) walks in nature, painting and drawing	volunteer work once a week, oriental dance once a week, Tibetan massage (twice a week)
2010	FTRE, PKV	(working at home) walks in nature, painting, and drawing	volunteer work once a week, occasional oriental dance at home, Tibetan massage (twice a week)

Most of the above activities have been discussed in other chapters of this book: visualizations, mirror work, the Phyllis Krystal method, etc.

Let me say a few words about the activities that have not been mentioned elsewhere in the book.

Walks in nature. This is my daily routine habit that I try to maintain regardless of the weather. Some days I prefer the forest by the river close to where I live. I call it a magical forest, since it is so quiet. All you can hear is the river, dry branches falling to the ground, and the beautiful songs of birds. The path is only reachable on foot, so there is no traffic.

If I have more energy I ascend a hill nearby and enjoy the great view of the town below and of the Alps in the distance. I walk past isolated farms, fields, forest patches, meadows, and pastures. Sometimes the sound of a farm tractor interrupts the silence, but most of the time it is quiet.

Despite the sublime beauty of my solitude in nature, on some days I prefer to take a walk towards the center of the town I live in. It is usually when I do not have any appointments. I work at home, so if I have no meetings, I start missing company a bit.

In other words: on one hand I yearn for a lonely walk after having been exposed to angry or complaining people for hours. On the other hand I look forward to meeting positive people in the town center.

Thus I somehow pursue a balance between being too social and not social enough by "taking different doses of solitude in nature".

Despite the three variations of my walks mentioned above, it might become a boring routine if I was not paying interest to details. I notice all kind of changes in nature: the level of the water in the river, the color of the leaves, the new blossoms, the color of clouds, the moods of the people passing by, etc.

There are some days when I do not want to go for a walk because I think I have to do some more work. I always regret it, for the next day I wake up with a headache. I could see my sensitive brain as my drawback, but I choose not to. I see it as a precious jewel enabling me to marvel at nature's beauty every day or to run into an acquaintance in the town center and have a nice chat.

How different from the winter and early spring of 2004, when I was so depressed that I would not even get out of bed the whole day. I remember struggling for hours to get myself up, put on my shoes, and go for a 10-minute walk. I think it was not even half a mile. I felt like a loser, because prior to the depression I had gone on some really long hikes and I had even run a 26-mile marathon in 2000. Yes, I felt like a real loser in 2004, when I was only able to walk for 10 minutes very slowly. But if I think about it today, it was not in vain. Every step counts. Whatever you do, never give up totally.

Volunteer work. I visit a lady at the local retirement home every Tuesday. I chat with her. We have become friends.

Incense burning and listening to soft instrumental music. Traditional Tibetan incense and calming music help me relax and stay focused on my Phyllis Krystal method visualizations. I also burn incense and drink calming Tibetan herb tea or chamomile tea in the evening when I am stressed out and I anticipate difficulties falling asleep.

AN OVERVIEW OF ALL
THE PERSONAL GROWTH SEMINARS
I HAVE TAKEN PART IN

November 1998 – September 2000, *Alternativna terapevtska skupnost dr. Janeza Ruglja* (Alternative Therapy Group of Janez Rugelj, PhD).

22 – 23 April 2006, Novo mesto, Slovenia, P. Krystal's seminar: *Cutting the Ties*.

3 – 4 November 2007, Ljubljana, Slovenia, P. Krystal's seminar: *Family Relationships and Communication* (first day). *Family Patterns* (second day).

15 – 16 December 2007, Aarau, Switzerland, P. Krystal's seminar: *Advanced Seminar of the Phyllis Krystal Method*.

16 October 2008 – 5th February 2009 (12 weekly sessions plus a weekend seminar), CDK – Šola čustvene inteligence (School for Emotional Intelligence), Ljubljana, Slovenia, B. Trtnik's seminar: *5 Steps to Better Relationships*.

29 – 30 November 2008, Ljubljana, Slovenia, P. Krystal's seminar: *Dreams* (first day). *Taming the Monkey Mind* (second day).

4 March – 3 June 2009 (12 weekly sessions), CDK – Šola čustvene inteligence (School for Emotional Intelligence), Ljubljana, Slovenia, L. Ivandič's seminar: *How to Handle Our Emotions I*.

27 – 29 March 2009, CDK – Šola čustvene inteligence (School for Emotional Intelligence), Kranjska Gora, Slovenia, N. Leskovar's weekend seminar: *The Power of Self-Trust*.

18 April 2009, Aarau, Switzerland, P. Krystal's seminar: *Live-Demo with Phyllis Krystal*.

15 – 17 and 22 – 24 May 2009 (two weekend seminars), Kope, Slovenia, T. Kalsang's seminar: *A Brief Introduction to Traditional Tibetan Medicine*.

4 – 7 March 2010, Munich, Germany, P. Krystal's seminar: *Phyllis Krystal Method Training Program, First Session*.

28 – 31 October 2010, Munich, Germany, P. Krystal's seminar: *Phyllis Krystal Method Training Program, Second Session*.

Glossary of Terms

affirmation – An affirmative sentence in the present tense, including only positive terms, intended to change our thinking patterns to more positive ones. For example, you affirm "I am *slim*." and not "I am not *fat*." One affirms things that will be true, but still uses the present tense. Affirmations are most effective if they are repeated aloud in front of a mirror while looking into one's eyes (*mirror work*). See L. Hay's books.

antipsychotic medication – Medication in the form of pills or injections that stabilizes one's mood and prevents or eliminates psychotic symptoms: delusions, hallucinations, paranoia, megalomaniacal ideas, and insomnia. Another term for this kind of medication is *neuroleptica*.

antipsychotic pills, see *antipsychotic medication*

bipolar disorder – A new term for manic-depression. See also *schizoaffective disorder* below.

CBT, see *cognitive-behavioral therapy*

cognitive-behavioral therapy – A type of psychotherapy which is used to help people change their thoughts, feelings, and behaviors that are causing them problems. See also *thinking patterns* below.

destigmatization – Refers to various ways of raising public awareness of mental illness in order to remove the *stigma* from it. *Stigma* entails the *shame* felt by those who have the illness and the *contempt* shown by those who know the mental patients. Such stigma also lowers the chances of getting a job, a life partner, etc.

episode – In this book you can find expressions such as *mental illness episode, schizoaffective disorder episode, SchAD episode*, and *psychotic episode*. In the context of this book they mean the same thing. A mental illness episode is like being struck by a physical illness. It is a period of time during which the symptoms of the mental illness are very severe.

imagery, see *visualization*

inner child – A psychological term. It usually stands for the playful aspect of our personality, on one hand, and for the painful memories from our childhood, on the other hand.

mental exercise – Any exercise that helps us improve our thinking patterns. The usual types of mental exercises are: repeating positive sentences (affirmations), imagining positive scenes (visualizations), having positive sentences written on walls, different types of yoga meditation, etc. See also ***thinking patterns*** below.

mental work, see *mental exercise*

mirror exercises, see *affirmation*

mirror work, see *affirmation*

Phyllis Krystal method – A method developed by Phyllis Krystal can help us cut the ties that bind us to anyone or anything that acts as an authority and exerts control over us. Detachment from such control will allow us to remove the accumulated layers of conditioning which obscure the inner light of the Higher Consciousness (Hi C) or Real Self. The exercises that are contained in this method can help to free us from everything that prevents the Real Self from being expressed through the exterior shell or receptacle comprising the body, mind, personality, and ego.

post-psychotic emptiness – The lack of energy and intense death wish that follows a mental illness episode (see *episode* above).

SchAD, see *schizoaffective disorder*

schizoaffective disorder – You can look up more professional definitions on the internet, but let me give you a very simplified version here. For me, *schizoaffective disorder – bipolar type* is a combination of **schizophrenia** and **bipolar disorder**. Bipolar disorder is called *bi*-polar, because it includes **both** *manic* (excessive happiness and self-worth feelings) and *depressive* (excessive sadness and emptiness) symptoms. Furthermore, *hallucinations, paranoia*, and other *delusions* are typical of schizophrenia. There are two types of schizoaffective disorder. There is the above mentioned bipolar type, and another one called depressive type. The second type lacks manic symptoms – that is the most important difference between the two types.

thinking patterns – Ways of thinking that affect your emotions, words, and deeds. If you manage to improve your ways of thinking, your emotions, words, and deeds will change for the better too. Let me give you an example. I have a thinking pattern called perfectionism, which means that I think that I have to be *perfect*. Since this is impossible, I am always disappointed. Then, through mental exercises I manage to change my thinking pattern to: "It is fine if I am *good enough*." That way I will approve of myself in most situations (*emotion*). I will say to myself "Well done." more often (*words*). And I will be more self-assured when taking action, for the fear of failure will be reduced (*emotion*). Consequently I will take more action and procrastinate less (*deeds*). See also **mental exercise** above.

visualization – A nice scene one imagines in order to calm down or to change one's thinking patterns into more positive ones. Visualizations are typical of yoga meditation, autogenic training (Western medicine approach), the Phyllis Krystal method, and many other approaches. Another word for this is *imagery*.

Endnotes

1. Hay, L. L., 2008 (1st printing 1984). *You Can Heal Your Life.* Carlsbad (CA, USA): Hay House.
2. Kelder, P., 1998 (1st printing 1985). *Ancient Secret of the Fountain of Youth.* Gig Harbor, Wash. (USA): Harbor Press.
3. Hay, L. L., 2008 (1st printing 1984). *You Can Heal Your Life.* Carlsbad (CA, USA): Hay House. Pages 72–73.
4. See: http://www.starchild.co.za/what.html . This text is based on an article by dr. Doreen Virtue.
5. See: http://www.starchild.co.za/what.html . This text is based on an article by dr. Doreen Virtue.
6. Hay, L. L., 2008 (1st printing 1984). *You Can Heal Your Life.* Carlsbad (CA, USA): Hay House.
7. McColl, P., 2007. *Your Destiny Switch. Master Your Key Emotions, and Attract the Life of Your Dreams!* USA: Hay House. Page 116.
8. See: http://www.starchild.co.za/what.html . This text is based on an article by dr. Doreen Virtue.
9. This is a term from Phyllis Krystal's terminology. See: Krystal, P., 1993. *Cutting More Ties that Bind. Letting Go of Fear, Anger, Guilt, and Jealousy so We Can Educate our Children and Change Ourselves.* Samuel Weiser: York Beach, Maine, USA. Pages 106–112.
10. This is a term from P. Krystal's terminology. See: Krystal, P., 1993. *Cutting more Ties that Bind. Letting Go of Fear, Anger, Guilt, and Jealousy so We Can Educate our Children and Change Ourselves.* Samuel Weiser: York Beach, Maine, USA. Pages 106–112.
11. Kalsang, T., 2009. *A Brief Introduction to Traditional Tibetan Medicine*, 15th–17th and 22nd–24th of May 2009, Kope, Slovenia.
12. McTaggart, L., 2008. *The Field – The Quest for the Secret Force of the Universe.* New York: Harper.
13. Ziglar, Z., 2008. *Inspiration. 365 Days A Year.* Naperville, Illinois, USA: Simple Truths. Page 51.
14. P. Krystal explained this particular point about children in an interview for the Slovene newspaper *Delo*, Supplement: *Ona*, article: *Zakaj ne poskusite z osmico?*, interviewed by: Lea Jelen, 27 January 2009, page 14.
15. Cutler, H. C. and His Holiness The Dalai Lama XIV, 1998. *The Art of Happiness. A Handbook for Living.* Chapter 14: Dealing with Anxiety and Building Self-Esteem. Riverhead Books.
16. See Wikipedia on www.
17. P. Krystal, Aufbauseminar – Phyllis Krystal Methode, 15th- 16th of December 2007, Kurszentrum Aarau, Switzerland.
18. H. C. Cutler and His Holiness The Dalai Lama XIV: *The Art of Happiness. A Handbook for Living.* Chapter 8: Facing Suffering. Pages 133 – 148. Riverhead Books: 1998.
19. Hay, L. L., 2008 (1st printing 1984). *You Can Heal Your Life.* Carlsbad (CA, USA): Hay House.
20. Hay, L. L., 1992. *The Power Is Within You.* Audio Book. Six-tape set. Carlsbad (CA, USA): Hay House.

Index

affirmations 36, 39, 60, 65, 85, 86, 93, 115, 116
alarm light 86
alternative medicine 87, 88, 89, 90, 93
antipsychotic medication VIII, 22, 72, 74, 83, 87, 88, 90, 96, 101
antipsychotic pills, *see antipsychotic medication*
anxiety 4, 12, 50, 51, 73, 88, 91
aura 45, 60, 65, 93
autosuggestion, *see self-programming*
biochemical irregularities 4, 5, 51, 69, 87, 88, 91, 108
bio-energy healer 35, 94
bipolar 4, 16, 17
bipolar disorder, *see bipolar*
catastrophic scenario 34, 36, 37
CBT, *see cognitive-behavioral therapy*
character 50, 51, 53, 54, 55, 59, 60, 61, 64
cognitive-behavioral therapy 90, 91, 92, 93, 96, 115
coincidence VIII, 23, 53, 63, 76, 77, 78, 107
colleagues at work 48, 102
concentration 12, 17, 18, 20, 24, 41, 52
delusions 11, 16, 33
denial 33, 34, 48, 87, 100
depression 12, 16, 17, 21, 22, 25, 30, 35, 39, 73, 91, 97, 117
depressive, *see depression*
destigmatization, *see stigma*
dopamine 51
early symptoms 101

episode VII, 11, 15, 18, 20, 21, 22, 29, 30, 33, 34, 35, 36, 38, 39, 49, 50, 69, 70, 84, 90, 95, 101, 103, 105, 111

everyone's savior 53, 54, 55, 57, 58

fear exercise 37

fear VIII, 5, 12, 14, 33, 34, 35, 37, 50, 53, 54, 60, 69, 70, 72, 74, 75, 76, 78, 88, 90, 95, 97

first date 103

five Tibetan rejuvenating exercises 28, 35, 115

friends 97, 98, 100, 117

genetic 62, 63, 64

good little girl 60

guilt 52, 53, 60, 95

habit 39, 64, 85, 92, 95, 96, 99, 104, 105, 107, 108, 116

hallucinations 14, 16, 18, 30, 33

humor 3, 100

imagery, *see visualizations*

indigo children 45, 46, 47, 49, 50

inner child 75

inner drives 56

insomnia 94, 95, 103

integrative medicine 87

job interview 102, 103

lifestyle 26, 88, 94, 95, 96

locked ward XI, 14, 30, 87, 101

manic VII, 11, 16, 17, 22, 101

manic-depressive VII, 12, 30

megalomaniacal ideas 23, 30

mental exercises 35, 36, 39, 58, 60, 64, 70, 75, 84, 85, 86, 88, 90, 94, 96, 98

mental work, *see mental exercises*

mirror exercises, *see affirmations*

mirror work, *see affirmations*
natural healing 88, 93, 96
negativity 99
paranoia, *see paranoid*
paranoid 12, 16, 18, 30, 33, 88
people pleaser 53, 54, 55, 56, 57, 58
people who live with us 100
perfectionism 53, 54, 60
personality traits 4, 45
Phyllis Krystal method 58, 60, 69, 70, 71, 75, 86, 93, 96, 115, 116, 117
positive thinking 38
post-psychotic emptiness 35
pre-menstrual syndrome 87, 91
principle of resistance 96
psychiatric clinic 14, 15, 24, 30, 33, 34, 35, 48, 49, 101
psychosis, *see psychotic*
psychotherapy 26, 28
psychotic XI, 11, 13, 15, 18, 21, 22, 30, 35, 36, 70, 84, 105
Reiki 93, 96
relatives 90, 98, 100
saying thanks 105
SchAD, *see schizoaffective disorder*
schizoaffective disorder 4, 5, 11, 16, 17, 18, 20, 21, 22, 29, 30, 33, 34, 38, 39, 47, 48, 49, 50, 54, 69, 70, 72, 73, 83, 87, 88, 89, 90, 91, 93, 94, 95, 101, 103, 111
schizophrenia 16, 93
school for emotional intelligence 52, 59, 86, 93
self-esteem 4, 26
self-image 26, 40, 50, 55, 56, 65
self-observation 100

self-pity 49, 84, 85
self-programming 93
self-reliance 55
situational fears 34
sleeping disorders 12, 33, 89, 95, 98
stigma XII, 3, 21, 28
submissive 53, 55, 59
submissiveness, *see submissive*
sugar 104
suicidal VII, XI, 4, 5, 17, 30, 85, 91, 97, 108
suicide, *see suicidal*
swamp and tractor 59
talk therapy 26, 28
talking total nonsense 12
thinking patterns VIII, 5, 58, 64, 85, 94, 104, 108
Traditional Tibetan Medicine 59, 94
Tri-pa energy 59
visualizations 36, 52, 58, 65, 69, 70, 77, 85, 86, 115, 116, 117
volunteer work 76, 115, 117
walks in nature 115, 116
watching TV 104
worry 4, 12, 34, 52, 53, 96

PRAISE FOR Balancing the Beast

"In my opinion, the book can help many people find a way to move forward." – **Klelija Hrovatič, MD, Psychiatrist**

"While Bipolar Disorder for Dummies is an encyclopedia of bipolar disorder, Helena Smole's book is a first-person story of a successful medical case." – **Professor Rok Tavčar, MD, PhD, Psychiatrist**, Head of the Rehabilitation Department, Psychiatric Clinic of Ljubljana

"The author definitely decided to switch her destiny to an optimistic mode and is more than willing to motivate other mental patients as well." – **Peggy McColl**, New York Times Best-Selling Author

"Many of my patients with mental illness often have difficulties with themselves. It is to them in particular that I would strongly recommend this book. It will help them to accept themselves, to face their illness, and to more easily live with it. The book contains a great amount of useful advice that can open up different possibilities for anyone. In addition, it is written in a very sincere manner, with a wealth of personal experience and invested effort.
I would recommend this book to anyone who is bothered by chronic illness or find themselves at the crossroads of life. Inspiring!" – **Lejla Doberšek**, MD, specialist in family medicine